TIME OUT *for a* KNEE REPLACEMENT

Between Faith Healing and Modern Medicine

MIRIAM MARANZENBOIM

Paperback ISBN: 978-1-64184-752-0
eBook ISBN: 978-1-64184-753-7

Back cover pictures: http://www.smithwigglesworth.com, http://newbirthminds.com, https://www.nytimes.com/2009/12/16/us/16roberts.html

Dem bones, dem bones, dem_dry bones
Now hear the word of [the Lord] [the surgeon]

4 There are [allotments or various kinds] diversities of gifts, but the same Spirit. 5 There are differences of ministries, but the same Lord. 6 And there are diversities of activities, but it is the same God who works [all things in] all in all. 7 But the manifestation of the Spirit is given to each one for the profit of all: 8 for to one is given the word of wisdom through the Spirit, to another the word of knowledge through the same Spirit, 9 to another faith by the same Spirit, to another **gifts of healings** by [NU one] the same Spirit, 10 to another the working of miracles, to another prophecy, to another discerning of spirits, to another different kinds of tongues, to another the interpretation of tongues. 11 But one and the same Spirit works all these things, distributing to each one individually as He wills.

Unity and Diversity in One Body

12 For as the body is one and has many members, but all the members of that one body, being many, are one body, so also is Christ. 13 For by one Spirit we were all baptized into one body—whether Jews or Greeks, whether slaves or free—and have all been made to drink [NU omits into] into one Spirit. 14 For in fact the body is not one member but many. 1 Corinthians 12:4-14 (NKJV)

(bold is mine)

Dedicated to Dan Bohi

TABLE OF CONTENTS

INTRODUCTION

The purpose of this book is three-fold. It seems that more and more people are doing knee replacements lately. I wish to encourage anyone who isn't convinced it's the solution for them that it's OK to do it. I'll be going into the details leading up to the actual surgery. Secondly, I feel that the scriptures which spoke to me during my recovery time are worth sharing. They will inspire you. In fact, just going over them yesterday and writing on each one, I realize how rich the Word of G-d is, and how I need to spend much more time reading it daily. Thirdly, I wish to share my journey which is as if on a path between the "faith-healing" side and the "professional medical side."

Since I've been living in Israel since 1977 and am used to writing G-d, instead of God (the religious folks do this out of respect), you will notice this and also that

I use the word "Yeshua" for Jesus, except for when you get to the scriptural comments chapter.

Miriam Maranzenboim

ABOUT BONES

Dem bones, dem bones, dem_dry bones

Dem bones, dem bones, dem_dry bones

Dem bones, dem bones, dem_dry bones

Now hear the Word of the Lord!

The foot bone connected to the ankle bone, the ankle bone connected to the leg bone, the leg bone connected to the knee bone, the knee bone connected to the thigh bone, the thigh bone, connected to the hip bone, the hip bone connected to the back bone, the back bone connected to the neck bone, the neck bone connected to the head bone, Now hear the word of the Lord.

This song goes way back to the early days when there was slave trade in the U.S.A.

Estimates are that about 12 million to 12.8 million Africans were shipped across the Atlantic over a span of 400 years. The Black folks, now referred to as "blacks" and not Negroes, would sing songs while working on the plantations. They worked long hours in cotton fields in the hot sun.

Don't worry readers, this book is not "woke"; out to blame the U.S.A. for the past. In our day and age we're hearing about how America was bad because of this. Well, do you know what Abraham Lincoln did? He emancipated them. Now after many years and the effort of such people as Martin L. King, Jr. they hold honorable places all over the country at many levels. The first black president, Barack Obama, was elected in 2009. This was unimaginable in the previous century.

There are lots of references in the Bible mentioning bones. We're familiar with the passage about the dry bones coming together; the house of Israel (Ezekiel 37). Some use this passage to mean other things. I say let's stick with the original meaning since that's in fact what's happening here. My husband and I have been living in Israel since the late 70's and it's not the same country any more. It's truly coming alive. The desert is becoming like a Garden of Eden. We are blessed despite the challenges of daily life here in this neighborhood of the world.

THE PATH BETWEEN TWO SIDES

I grew up attending a typical active evangelical church in Rosemead, California. We were a family of four and we all knew the Word of G-d. We also memorized scripture. We heard sermons from our pastors and from all of the "right" visitors (from the "right" seminaries). When the Torchbearers of Capernwray came through from England I took special note and was hooked. I attended their Bible school for a few months and saved ALL of my notes from there for more than fifty years! During the covid-19 period I typed them up and now my Capernwray books (volume one and two) are for sale on amazon.

My sister had a "different" sort of boyfriend in high school. He was Pentecostal. This was the first time I encountered someone from that denomination. She also had a girlfriend who was from a so-called "charismatic" church. This girl made an impression and we actually held a Good News Club in her home. Then in my college years I came across the ministry of "Tia Linda" ("Tia" is "aunt" in Spanish) through a radio program. She needed some visual aids for her children's crusades in Spanish-speaking countries. I gladly took the "over-sized" flannel graph figures which she gave me and although I'm not an artist, I glued them on backgrounds I had drawn since she was teaching children outdoors. I put glue over them for preservation. When she flew to her assignment, these visual aids were kept in the cockpit of the plane. I'm sorry to say that they "somewhat" stuck together due to the humidity in those areas. I hope something was useful. I admired this single woman who could teach huge crowds of children in Spanish. There was a certain dimension in her faith which I seemed to lack. You guessed it – leaning to Pentecostalism or outright, I'm not sure.

I was in Europe for an entire year from 1965-66. After attending Capernwray, my parents told me about a three-month Child Evangelism Fellowship training course to be held in France (in the English language). Of course, I was interested. They would pay my bills to attend. A couple of classmates invited me to join them. They told me they prayed in tongues. I told them that when I received the Holy Spirit I received all of Him. I wasn't interested.

Back in the U.S.A. I had to decide what to do in life. I attended Biola College for a semester and then transferred to Multnomah School of the Bible in Portland. My sister attended this college for the entire four years. In both of these schools there was no mention of these Pentecostal phenomena.

Fast forward to 1977 when my former "fireman" boyfriend wanted to do volunteer work in Israel. I thought this sounded very interesting. We had cheap tickets via a university (I was a part-time student and could qualify). We ended up near Afula and found kibbutz life challenging, especially due to Israel's very hot summers. I was already past age thirty. The Hebrew class in the evening was not impressive. Two girls opted out and went to another kibbutz. I asked the director if he could find me a more serious framework for learning Hebrew. He found a place for me at Kibbutz Yad Mordechai ("yad" means hand in Hebrew) near Ashkelon. It was a great program; namely, four hours of Hebrew study per day and four hours of work. This varied every other week, whether morning or afternoon studies. I began to learn Hebrew with gusto. We were only about twenty students and from various countries. Not all of them were enthusiastic workers, I'm sorry to say. Being young, some would stay up late listening to music (bothersome!) and had a hard time getting up very early to work. Some reported that they were ill. It's very hot in the summer and one needs to be out in the field as early as 4 a.m. in order to finish early. There were dropouts as the weeks passed. Instead of three girls in my room, we went down to two. Shulamit, my roommate, was an Iranian Jewess who joined us later in the program. She had to flee from there since she was the postal manager's secretary and could no longer hide her Jewish identity. She was clever at picking up Hebrew and even obtained a Hebrew typewriter and began to type. Some of the students had family in Israel and would visit them on the weekends. Others simply rested or went various places, despite a lack of public bus service on Sabbath. I happily stayed in my room alone on Sabbath and chose to fast. I would learn the Hebrew words from the previous week and perhaps catch up on some hand wash. I could also sleep in which was, no doubt needed. This wonderful five-month course made all the difference for my future years in Israel. I left speaking conversational Hebrew.

I knew I needed to get to Jerusalem after this course since I had only limited contact with believers in Yeshua (the Hebrew name for Jesus) during these months in Israel. In the other part of this book I use "Jesus" since I'm using many Bible quotes. At first I stayed in a youth hostel in the Old City of Jerusalem. I had temporary jobs typing English but what would be long-term? I had very few possessions. It was very rainy and one needs boots since you're bussing and have to stand outside sometimes in pouring rain (of course with an umbrella!). I bought my first pair of boots. It was a particularly rainy winter in 1966. By the Lord's amazing providence I came across a group called the Mount Zion Fellowship. Sister Ruth Heflin and Sister Susan Woodaman (from an unsaved military family) were in charge of a group of around twenty folks from various countries, but mostly Americans. The Pentecostals referred to one another as "Brother" and "Sister."

These leaders lived in an impressive Arabic-style "mansion" (we called it the "big house") next to the British Consulate in the wealthy area of east Jerusalem called Sheikh Jarrah. Yes, you HAVE heard about it lately in the news. They're fighting over property; Jews vs. Arabs. I would never have imagined that this place where I was able to live would show up big time forty years later. The rest of the folks lived in apartments in various places around town, both in the Jewish and Arab sectors. I was invited to their Christmas party. They had a big tree and invited the Orthodox priests from the Old City and various other folks (probably mostly English-speaking).

I was like an orphan on the doorstep but they took a chance and invited me to actually live with them. I asked how much it would cost. I suppose they laughed. They said that I would need to attend their evening services on Friday, Saturday and Sunday evenings. Then there were the four-hour prayer meetings on Friday and Saturday mornings. I surely needed an arrangement like this. The "price" was right. Here was where I began to understand for the first time something about

Pentecostals. They would come into the rented church called "St. Peter in Gallicantu" ("gallicantu" is rooster in Italian) and stand and pray or sing in tongues moving their hands upward and down for a few minutes before the service. We always started promptly at 7 p.m. I liked this part – also the finishing on time. Sister Ruth Heflin used to say that the Holy Spirit could say everything He needed to say within that time. I say "Amen" and wish other groups would adopt this. One evening someone gave a prophetic word and a Russian-speaking person entered the room right at that moment and could translate it for us. We see this in 1 Corinthians 14. I simply sat there and read this chapter while watching others in the beginning. For the first time I understood the difference between tongues and prophecies. There's a place and time for each. It doesn't have to be complicated. I was hungry for more of G-d. I received the gift of tongues but I didn't experience any "touch" from G-d. Sister Susan came to me. I was encouraged just to open my mouth and speak what seemed to be gibberish but this is the language I still pray in sometimes. The idea is simply to get out of our natural "mind-set." When we're using our reasoning too much G-d can't get past and do anything. We're to "go higher." I mean that if I'm praying for an individual I don't need to worry about the words. When we pray in tongues G-d hears and sorts it all out and does something in that person's life. I'm not smart enough to know their specific needs, correct? If

G-d puts a person suddenly into my thoughts, I simply pray for them at that moment.

This group believed in G-d's healing power. If someone cut their hand I don't think they even kept a box of band aids in their house. They would pray. I trusted G-d to heal my eyes and didn't wear glasses for a while. The muscles were strengthened, but I did go back to the glasses afterwards. We did lots of fasting. I was on a spiritual high. Food became less important for me. One Saturday morning at the little chapel near Bethlehem they prayed for a husband for me. Can you imagine this? Bara and Burt prayed and I met Michael the following week! Burt has since gone to be with the Lord. When I met people and told them this, they asked, "Where ARE those folks?" Funny. G-d was very good to me. I count my blessings daily. Michael and I have been married for more than 42 years. We have 4 children and 14 grandchildren in the meantime. I owe the Mt. Zion Fellowship a great debt of gratitude. They even enabled me to attended Hebrew University. I studied at both campuses. Somehow there was money for the tuition. My grades at the end of my university days left something to be desired. I studied Hebrew but ended up in the wrong level; my fault. The courses in the history of the Jewish people and the history of Israel were very valuable. I kept the notes I took until today. I even typed up part of them for the next generation (hoping they'll look at them!). Both Sister Ruth and Sister Susan would travel to exotic places in their lifetime, such as Tibet and China. They saw G-d's miracles, including healings. They've both written books which are obtainable. Considering how much we fasted, it was surprising how the group remained healthy. I stayed with them for about two years and don't remember anyone becoming ill.

MOVING TO THE GALILEE

Michael and were married abroad. His congregation in Haifa gave us a nice reception shortly after we returned to Israel. Rose Warmer (a Jewess with a remarkable testimony; she wrote a book) donated five cakes to the event. I doubt if we finished them since there weren't very many people in attendance. My fellowship in Jerusalem also had a reception for us. The layer cake was very impressive. Sister Ruth loved weddings. Others followed after ours. Michael thankfully "flowed" with the Pentecostal flavor of the group.

Michael and I settled into his bachelor apartment in Migdal HaEmek. After less than six months someone in the interior ministry gave us a two-bedroom apartment on the 4th floor in which we lived for many years. We were even able to purchase it at a discount price since we'd lived in it consistently. We'd only paid a short visit to my folks and friends in California when our first two children were under age two (it was cheap for them).

Raising four children in an apartment on the 4th floor, I encountered back problems from time to time. I remember my parents would also experience a "slipped disc." When they did, they went to their osteopath to get treated. When I had back pain there were two people who helped. One was a religious gal who was a physiotherapist. She had the special table in her home and I could walk there for treatment. On another occasion or two, a Frenchman came to our apartment. I needed to be on our dining room table. He had a lamp – I suppose it was heat. The children would see me on the table! I think he massaged my back, if I remember correctly. It helped.

Only in 1991 when we heard about the ICEJ (International Christian Embassy in Jerusalem) Feast of Tabernacles did we encounter healing meetings. I found out in time that the Assemblies of G-d denomination teaches the five-fold ministries, healing, tongues and prophecies. During the feast there's not "super" evidence of these things which is OK. I would sometimes hear the people in the evening service in the main auditorium singing in tongues for about five minutes. Then they would stop. It was beautiful. The embassy folks are very solid with the Word of G-d which is important. They drew thousands of folks from all over the world for many, many years. My husband attended with our family for about the first four years. He would go from healing meeting to healing meeting. It interested him. The first year we attended Martie Haaijer's healing meeting at the YMCA. I had back problems and I went forward for healing. The attendants prayed for me and I fell backwards but someone catches you. After this I didn't have the monthly back pain. The pain had originated long before coming to Israel since I lifted a "too heavy" color TV into the back of my car to take to my folk's place. I suppose we intended to watch something special.

Even after this "healing" I would have back pain from time to time. Sometimes we move incorrectly. Maybe we lift something we shouldn't. I heard about an alternative chiropractor on a kibbutz near Midgal HaEmek and went to him a number of times. I also recommended him to others; even taking someone to him in my car one or more times. He always did "hands on" treatment and it always helped. He had so many clients that he needed to get an assistant. Once I went to the assistant. The pain was relieved. I have to mention these treatments since I'm talking about "faith healing" (yes, I've experienced it!), but that it's also OK to go to these professionals when we need to. Remember we can also testify to them, which I do.

When I was pregnant with the four children I developed varicose veins. I had to wear support hosiery which my mother would send from the USA. Once I needed to shop with my daughter for a white blouse for a special event. I had such pain that I needed to sit down. I told her to go alone and find one. I continued to attend the Feast of Tabernacles with the children year after year. It was our "family vacation." There was a healing meeting on a Friday afternoon with Christine Darg. She spoke and prayed. She mentioned someone with varicose veins. I was standing and the pain went away at that moment. After this I was fine for years. In time, however, it became worse. My mother had varicose veins. The solution was to operate. I had the vein strip surgery on one leg and never had any problem after this. The Lord gave me my second book during the recovery time when I needed to keep the legs elevated in bed. I wrote about it in *Two Books for Daniel.* The inspiration was a CD with messages on Daniel by W.A. Criswell which a boarder left behind. Later he couldn't remember who had given it to him. It opened a huge door for me. After Yeshua, Daniel is my favorite biblical character.

While we were living in Midgal HaEmek (more than 30 years!), I would swim at Nahalal, the Moshav ("communal" except land and home ownership) of "Moshe Dayan" fame. Sometimes I would swim in the ocean during the summer since two beaches near my work places in Haifa were without waves.

We moved to Haifa in 2009. Now I could swim very near our apartment at the famous Leo Baeck sports center. I also participated in the gym classes such as Feldenkrais and pilates. There were organized trips for the seniors monthly. They were well-planned and I thoroughly enjoyed them. Michael also joined us at times. Our age creeps up on us. My knees began bothering me. I went to an orthopedic surgeon; a specialist on knees. He said he could give me three injections, one or two weeks apart (can't remember). I bought them at the high price of 700+ NIS.

A few days after buying them I met a nice person from the USA who bought my book, "Josephus – The History of the Jews Condensed in Simple English" at the annual picnic of the Galilee where I had my sale table. This fellow contacted me via cellphone the following day and said that since he was still in Haifa he wanted me to sign his copy of the book. No problem. He came over and met us (my husband too). In our conversation we found out he was a VIP who was part Jewish and hoping to make Aliyah ("Aliyah", meaning in Hebrew, "going up," is the phenomena of diaspora Jews coming home to Israel). We were amazed that he had become a Messianic Jew. He mentioned that he had visited Kathryn Kuhlman's healing meetings years ago before he was saved. Well, I'd also visited her meetings. At the end of our conversation I asked if he could pray for my knees. He asked, "Do you have anointing oil?" What an amazing question. I went to get mine. I also pray for people and use my oil. After his prayer I did feel an improvement, so much so that I didn't need to use those injections. I tried for a long time to sell them online but no one even asked about them. More than one year passed. I continued swimming, walking and all. But we aren't getting any younger, correct? I went to the same orthopedic surgeon and he injected all three doses at once into my knee (they hadn't expired!). This helped for perhaps half a year.

Then the covid-19 arrived. The swimming pools were all closed. I would take a couple of walks per day in the neighborhood. I also kept up with some floor exercises most days. Months went by and we finally heard the exciting news that the pools would reopen. I ran into two people on the same day in a miraculous way who told me that Leo Baeck's pool would not reopen. I was prompted by the Holy Spirit to go to the Sportan in Haifa. They said they had a special price for those who had previously swam at Leo Baeck and that it would terminate by the weekend. I had no time to check out other options. I had peace about it, however, and signed up. We would need a vaccine but I didn't think twice. Swimming is important for my health. I also checked with my daughter since she's a pharmacist. She encouraged me to have the vaccine. I've had two so far since that's the requirement for pool entrance. I was back to swimming even as many as twelve lengths of the pool (times 25 meters). My knees weren't improving, however. Time came to have an x-ray. My knees are both bad but one was already bone-on-bone. The option was to operate.

PREPARING FOR THE OPERATION

I went to the surgeon who had given me the injection. He recommended the knee replacement surgery but he no longer performed them. He gave me the name of someone on the Carmel. I phoned and the secretary said it would cost 4,000 NIS. I did not make an appointment with this surgeon. I went to the office of Maccabi. This is the name of one of the four medical plans in Israel. I had switched from Clalit ("General") to Maccabi some years ago and was satisfied. My husband switched more recently. I asked at the office which orthopedic surgeon does knee replacements. I got a name and made an appointment. The bus stop was quite far from his office which was hidden in the midst of car garages, furniture stores, and "you name it" (Haifa's famous "Check Post" – a war-time name). My knees were hurting but I made it with the help of my map (I don't have a Smart phone!) and a couple of people along the way. The surgeon knew perfect English and explained how the operation would be done and showed me the plastic and metal "hinge" which would be put into my knee. The pictures here, which I took on my second and last visit to him show a reflection of my camera, my red/white dress and also of the surgeon's mask which he's wearing. They do a frontal cut. I asked, "What about the knee cap?" He said they move the patella ASIDE. OK… I don't need to know anything more. Young and efficient, he'd done internship in Canada. He said the operation wouldn't cost me anything. This was very important to hear! My vein strip operation had also been covered by Maccabi. I told him my husband's brother lived there and we'd visited. I said I didn't like it because it reminded me of Mexico. If

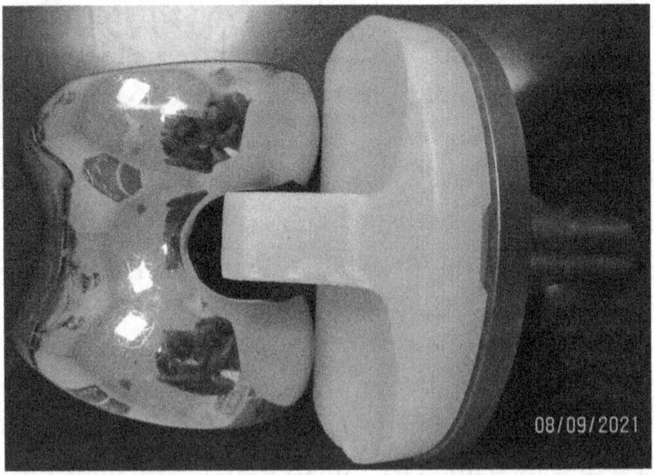

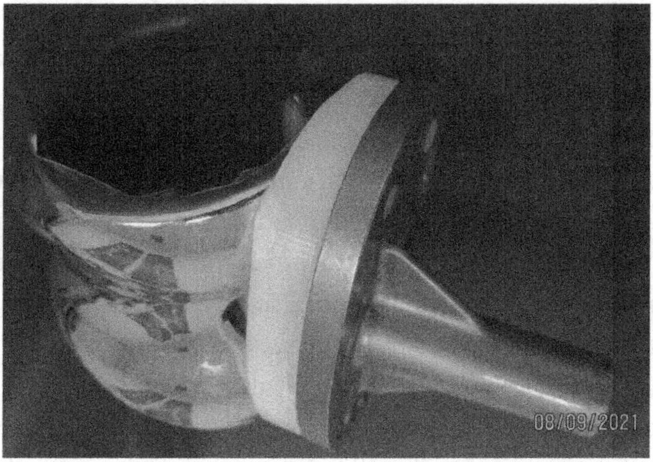

any Canadians are reading this they'd be insulted. There are beautiful parts in Toronto, of course. Just so happens that where Alfred was we'd walk in close proximity to his apartment and see within one glance five money exchange places. It was clearly a melting pot, including many Asians. The place where I could use a computer (VERY IMPORTANT FOR ME!) was run by an Asian and was filthy.

A number of people were waiting for this surgeon as I left. He IS in the right location since he's in walking distance of the Assuta Hospital of Haifa.

The operation was scheduled and I needed to arrive at the Assuta Hospital three days before that date. It's located within a Mall called "Lev HaMifratz" or "Heart of the Bay." I had my blood tests, disc with the chest x-ray (includes written explanation), stool test results, and my own printout from the blood tests. Of great importance was my Maccabi medical card. Research "Maccabi" – an important word. The sports teams are also Maccabi. With all of these I ASSUMED that I wouldn't need my "Teudat Zehut" which is our all-important identity card in Israel. Every place you phone for any type of service you're asked for this number. You also need this in order to vote (America has sorely missed on this point!). It has our picture on it, of course. I also didn't know that I needed an EKG. They explained that this was routine. As for the missing Teudat Zehut, the clerk even called the hospital director. The answer was that I must have it, otherwise there's NOTHING to do. Thankfully I have two sons living in Haifa. Rather than to have to go home via buses which is very time-consuming, I phoned a wonderful son who was willing to travel to my apartment, get the document and bring it to me. I have a book on kindle to read wherever I go, so I sat outside the hospital on the same floor waiting. In the thick of the traffic of the 3rd largest city in Israel, he jumped on his motorcycle and he showed up within one hour. To this day I felt very badly and prayed a lot for his safety. G-d had mercy on me since I could still see the anesthesiologist despite my failure. She took blood in order to know my type as well as a picture of my identity card. Both papers were put into a plastic envelope with "danger" written on it. This would go to the operating room I later found out! Of course, they need to be sure they have the right person and right blood type. Blood type has to be known in case of emergency (not that I needed any PTL). Her prick on my right inner elbow was awful. Blood oozed and I had a purple sign for days. It was the worst in 74 years! Think of giving birth to 4 children and how many times one needs these tests.

On the following day I went to do the EKG at the clinic. I ran into my husband there who was buying a new blood pressure machine. Ours was old. We could use my credit card. He doesn't have one so this was great timing. We've always tried to live "simply!" The next day I needed to buy birthday cards for Michael and Yoni in anticipation of being in hospital for weeks. I found them without too much walking in the Haifa Mall. My knees were bothering me at the time. If I hadn't written this down, I most surely would have forgotten. I should mention that many people are taking a substance called glucosamine sulfate in order to relieve the "bone-on-bone" sensation. I was taking this for years but in my case it wasn't helpful. I still take it for the non-operated leg. Norwegians and Swedes have bone issues in general. My mother's side was Swedish and her aunts all had "bandy legs" (bowed).

THE OPERATION DAY ARRIVED

Michael and I left for the hospital at 1:45 p.m. via the bus, then the Metronit (the double busses). My appointment was at 3 p.m. I needed to see the anesthesiologist first. She needed to see the EKG. She explained the options. I chose to do the "under-waist" plus another anesthesia to block pain in the knee area. I could've asked about this beforehand – like to have asked my son-in-law who is a surgeon. I simply decided since there's no time for anything. Then I talked with a nurse. She escorted us to my room and I put my things in the cupboard. When the time came it was all clothes off except the robe. There was a strange looking thing. I ignored it. I get to the location and they ask where my hat is. That "strange looking thing" was the cap which needed to be unfolded! The operation took place finally from 6 – 8 p.m. I KNOW that the waiting time can be nerve-wracking and I won't simply stare at a ceiling. I had *Trusting Him* by a former student of Temple City High School (my alma mater), Robert A. Boomsma, with me. He was married to a graduate from my year of 1964, but graduated one year later. His book is 540 pp. long and I insisted on having it with me. My insistence worked. Even when they wheeled me in they promised me that it would be on the bed upon coming out of surgery. This was an amazing book and I'm the only one who wrote a review on it so far. I just heard about the status of his health yesterday. Sad things, but he's pressing through. He's back home after serious surgeries but I encouraged him and am praying that the latest cancerous discovery will be healed by our Healer. He's been through enough. He does give credit to G-d for various miracles along the way in the past four months.

Michael took my hearing aids and glasses before I was wheeled in, and finally left after 8:30 p.m. I'm sorry he stuck around so long. He brought them back to me the next day. I didn't sleep a wink the first night and asked for pain pills MAXIMUM. My pharmacist daughter told me not to hesitate to request the meds BEFORE the severe pain begins. I could read with a night light and I already read 238 pp. of the book. Since I had to fast from 7 a.m. until the operation at 6 p.m., I had an appetite and asked for something to eat. They gave me two dairy products to eat in the middle of the night. Breakfast finally came before 8 a.m. I didn't leave a crumb. The coffee was perfect. I already took a couple of steps. Lunch – lovely. Read in the afternoon. Sleep evaded me. Someone came with a menu and asked which main entre we would like for dinner! It was "over" – I mean LOTS, since it was Sabbath. Two meat balls – I ate one and not all of the potatoes. Cold beets – yeah! This is Michael and my "magic" daily supper food. Carrots – too much pepper. Sweet potatoes and squash grilled (one of my favorite picks at an Israeli wedding – they overdo it with FOOD but each one pays so usually the bride and groom come out ahead). Chocolate on waffle for dessert. At 8 p.m. I had a narcotic pill, Percoset. Understand that for the first two weeks after this major operation one MUST take narcotic meds. The surgeon warned me about the pain. It's a more painful recovery than the hip replacement.

They bring a bed pan but after having that anesthesia, it's "frozen" there and nothing emerges, so no choice but a catheter. Finally it began after the catheter was taken out and it burned. The third time I needed the bed pan (we had to call the nurse to bring it!) I had an accident in the bed. I felt very badly and the nurse scolded me as if I did it on purpose. I told her it wasn't nice. She had to empty my pan three times. Perhaps this should've been a consideration when choosing the Anesthesiology (?). Someone reading this; take heed. I got Optalgin – 2 pills and liquid. I had to drink plenty of water. I already told the morning nurse I needed to shower and to sit on a toilet. Of course, I was VERY happy when the bed could be changed in the morning (at night I made due with a dry sheet folded in the needed place). Had a good morning. The next day I had a BM on the toilet, then shower. Sorry I write this but the entire book is about an operation, right? When we were post-delivery of a baby in the hospital they were concerned that we don't go home before having a BM. I wonder if they still do this. It's logical actually since they have things to help in case of difficulty. Now I was able to sit in a chair with my legs up. I was a new person but taking narcotics for the severe pain. Same breakfast as day before.

G-d and I made a deal before the operation that this would be an intimate time with Him. I'd be away from the hours and hours on my computer at home. I had a listening ear. The breakfast included granola to which one could add yoghurt (no milk). I had avoided eating granola for years since I thought I had sensitivity to oats. Israeli breakfasts include tomatoes and cucumbers. You add cottage cheese to them or eat the three different dairy products separately. The roll was nice. We had a hard-boiled egg and an apple. I ate EVERYTHING. I had no ill effects from that granola. My third son, Omer, phoned me from Germany. This was wonderful. One of the Sarah's (daughters-in-law) and Esther, my daughter, also phoned. I took a sleeping pill and slept for the first time that night. On the third day after surgery I was getting up more to the bathroom but groggy from pills. The breakfast was the same except that instead of the granola we had Telma corn flakes. I had never bought this brand of corn flakes since I thought I was sensitive to it. I ate everything; no ill effects. For lunch there was fish. In the evening "artificial" shawarma but it was OK. Good salad, soup and two dairy products. Assuta is a GOOD hospital. There are three branches in Israel. After four nights there I was moved to the Italian hospital for further recovery. Shai, mentioned before, came so I wouldn't be alone in the ambulance. Maccabi sent an SMS to my simple cellphone telling me that the cost of moving me in the MADA (Magen David Adom – similar to Red Cross) ambulance was covered.

TWO WEEKS OF RECOVERY AT THE ITALIAN HOSPITAL

The Italian Hospital is a beautiful, old style hospital with Spanish tile roof. From the upper floors at the back one had an exquisite view of Haifa Bay. There are very interesting pictures on the walls at the entrance, something like a museum. We enjoyed the beautiful living plants which lined the hallway downstairs and well-tended gardens outside. In time we'll be taking an elevator and walking outside without needing to step down, and walking along nice paths. There are enough benches to sit outside with our guests and we did this. It was an unusually cool June and we didn't need the air conditioner at night. Sea breezes entered our windows at night. We had a nice view of the green grass outside and very tall trees. You can google Italian Hospital, Haifa.

My roommate could hardly speak Hebrew. Her daughter was a newcomer from Moscow and coming to see her mother daily. She was studying Hebrew but didn't know very many words yet. I didn't write about the first week here except to say that I had a few visitors. The most joyful time was when my daughter-in-law came with the two girls. One brought her piano books so I could assign her what to play. I got to see pictures of the son's 13th birthday and this was special. The other daughter-in-law stopped by after work. It's OK that grandchildren don't come; it's sort of depressing to see folks in the hospital and we were in covid-19 time.

I have to mention the first supper I had in the English hospital. I saw half of a beautiful avocado on the plate. I haven't eaten them for years. I was curious about the liquid inside the hole of the avocado. It was lemon juice. I ate that avocado with gusto because of those previous breakfast incidents. Now without a doubt, I could see that G-d has a sense of humor. I had made a deal and He removed ALL of my dietary quirks within the first three days one after the other! This was cause for rejoicing. Back home I've switched to eating non-sweetened granola most mornings, together with yoghurt and some corn flakes or rice krispies (made in our former town, Migdal HaEmek!), and a tablespoon of honey. I've eaten avocados also.

Michael was visiting me almost every day between caring for his clients. He's been a caregiver for years and has a way with the old folks. I could have recovered in a place called "House in the Heart" or (Beit BeLev) in Nesher but I chose the Italian hospital since it would be closer to where he needed to be in the daytime. The surgeon had said that post-knee and hip surgery patients were satisfied with the care there. For years the Italian Hospital had the reputation of being for the dying folks. No more. They have two orthopedic departments for those recovering from hip or knee surgery – also from accidents. Michael brought me a few items which I'd forgotten to bring and also helped with washing some clothing items and returning them.

The nurses and staff were very gracious. From experience they knew better than to challenge any of us if we asked for medicine against pain. They showed up every time when we put the light on, including in the middle of the night. They would have to take our temperatures at 5 a.m. in the morning in order to be free for the big breakfast-time rush. We had to be showered and beds made BEFORE breakfast but they managed. They also had to bandage our legs from the ankle area up the upper leg to prevent thrombosis. They were very good at this and then they made sure the bandages were taken off at bedtime.

After one week of eating the well-prepared healthy food, I had a serious dilemma. When I asked for a remedy for constipation, they brought two very small glycerine-type items. The medicine is supposed to "work on you." No success. I phoned two former nurses that I know (one, a relative!). "Can you come and give me an enema?" They thought I was out of my mind but I was serious. One had been a clinical nurse and apparently had no experience with this. The other said, "They're dangerous – we don't do those anymore." What? Thankfully my children only needed one once if I recall but I did what needed to be done like my mother had to do for me. Water always worked. I well remember my Swedish grandmother's reaction to hearing if my sister or I were ill. She immediately said, "Give them a physic!" (an enema). (She was the only grandparent who was alive when I was born. How rich are my 14 grandchildren to have ALL of their grandparents alive at this writing?). What's dangerous about giving someone an enema with water, pray tell? Michael and I had a simple enema device at our apartment – a rubber ball which you'd fill with water, then press, and presto – it's inside. You cover the plastic insertion part with Vaseline so you don't hurt yourself when inserting. I told the nurses earlier in the morning that I was ON STRIKE. I wouldn't do ANYTHING until I had this problem solved! I phoned Michael and told him where I thought the gadget was at home. G-d heard me and helped him find it. PTL Michael was able to bring it same day and the device solved my problem. I was now a normal human being as opposed to one filled up with poison. If ever you think someone

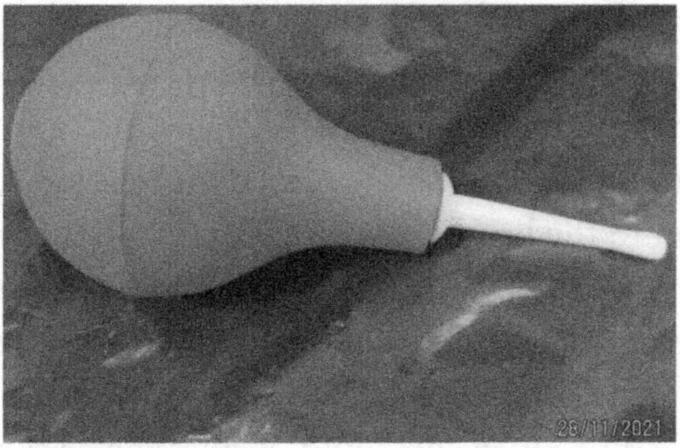

would commit suicide over this basic human problem, I could easily identify with them. BTW, it wasn't that the food wasn't what we needed; it was the narcotic pills which cause backup.

While we're on this delicate subject, I have to tell about a teenager in my building. She had a hemorrhoid operation. All of the suffering and missing days of school could've been avoided. I was very sad to hear about this. I blame her mother.

By now I had finished reading the 540 page book and began reading volume 4 by Lynn Austin, *Faith of My Father*.

June 11 (remember the surgery was May 27th) I was up to restroom at least three times during the night but otherwise slept well with pain med and the sleeping pill. Optalgin liquid at 6:30 a.m. since it can be taken without food. Otherwise we'd get our narcotic meds with breakfast. One problem was that the evening meal was served even BEFORE 6 p.m. and there's that long stretch at night until the 8 a.m. breakfast. No possibility for narcotic med in between. Michael brought me two grapefruits which was very nice; a morning "booster" in addition to the breakfast.

I didn't mention that the first roommate left after about 3 nights (I didn't write it down). I had a new bona fide Israeli roommate who insisted I speak Hebrew! This was fine since she could correct me at times. She got a technician to get the TV operating in the room. This was great – you'll understand in a few sentences down. Nurit liked coffee in the morning like I do. We would rise early and take a walk with our "walkers" before breakfast to the 3rd floor where they had boiling water. The cleaning lady was already working on our floor and saw us at this early hour and didn't like this idea. In fact, not everyone up on 3rd was pleased either. They found a remedy for us. They brought a water machine to the second floor, but the water was foul-tasting. We also needed to fill up our cold water bottles for the day. We continued on our early morning adventures. Once the double doors upstairs were closed. She exerted her strength and opened them. This is Israeli! We got our coffee and my milk was spoiled; I could use hers.

After a while she started reading her books. I realized we didn't really have too much to talk about. She and her husband had been ambassadors in a foreign country when their children were small. I felt like since she had since divorced, things were very different for her. Her daughter came to visit often and was clearly as spoiled as she was. I pray for various ones I met there even as I'm writing about them.

I finished all three Lynn Austin books in the series called Chronicles of the Kings. She's a historical fiction writer based on the Bible. I had read volumes one and two years ago; now I'd completed 3-5. She's a favorite. It could be that I read one of the latter books already on my kindle, this is OK…

This is what I wrote about one of the books: "They'd escaped Manasseh's cruelty and bringing in of false gods and established Jewish life, including temple on Elephantine Island. They brought the ark with them with a "disguised model."They also disguised themselves when necessary even if it meant shaving beard hair. Miriam warned Joshua that they would kill him but she fell in doing so and almost died. She's on crutches now but she ends up marrying Joshua. She lost both babies. Successor to throne of Manasseh would've been via Amariah. Joshua's adopted son Nathan and he are in Hezekiah's tunnel in the water. Joshua finally learns to forgive. Manasseh changes into a true worshipper of G-d in the end. There were quite a few illegitimate children in the story. Wars, wounded. Joshua's eye was injured – Hadad gets killed. He was jealous since a rival married Yael." It's not nice to give away plots but I do hope someone will read her books since there are TRUE elements in them from history. This is NOT the Joshua of the book of Joshua. I don't think I realized that the evil king Manasseh actually did have a change of heart at the end of his life until I read this book.

We went to physiotherapy daily except for Saturday when they were closed. On June 11 they gave me a walking stick. Up to now we were using walkers. The therapists are both native Arabic-speakers but knew Hebrew and English well. Sometimes they would put on what I call "high class" music – like the great Italian singers. One had attended medical school in Italy, the other in Spain. They didn't succeed but they were great therapists and used their good spirits and humor to get us to "work." Physiotherapy is the most important key to a successful recovery from both the knee and the hip replacement operations. One must be faithful, particularly when it comes to the knee flexibility. Sometimes you feel like you've taken two steps forward, later to feel like you've gone backwards by one step. This is normal. There were two wooden steps "up" in the room and we were stepping up already in the first week. One of the therapists would force my leg to bend better, to which I reacted with some sound. To this day, almost six months after surgery, I can't bend the operated knee more than 100 degrees – the right leg maybe bends 120. The surgeon visited us at least once in this facility. My doctor looked like a cowboy (plaid shirt, appropriate belt), and I said that he was just missing the hat. At a latter visit I learned that he has (is it?) five children?

A dear woman from the congregation visited and brought some goodies. It was nice of her. Her husband also visited Michael when he had abdominal surgery years ago. This was a true effort since he was working and later had to drive a great distance to the Afula hospital. He also visited Michael when he was at home when we lived in Migdal HaEmek. You don't forget the love and care of these folks. It's not surprising now that at their age that they're continuing to bless people through a particular congregation which is reaching out to the needy; food and clothing.

During the painful times in the hospital I actually read a total of six books before reading my New Testament. I read *Well Versed: Biblical Answers to Today's Tough Issues*, by Dr. James Garlow, *In, But Not Of: A Guide to Christian Ambition and the Desire to Influence the World* by Hugh Hewitt (2012) and up to Revelation 10 in the New Testament. I didn't comment on the New Testament verses after the first few notes I made of references in Romans. I mention these other books since I highly recommend them.

On June 10th Israel was being attacked. We were in the midst of changing prime ministers. There was lots of talk about former Prime Minister Begin. It was nice to be able to watch the news on our TV at 8 p.m. We closed the door since my roommate wanted to watch the music contests after the news. We did this for about 2-3 days. Since we don't have TV at home, I was exposed to what people devour 365 days of the year. I can do without most of it. I was thankful, however, to be able to see the swearing-in ceremony for Prime Minister Naftali Bennett on the 13th of June, 2021 and all of the 120 new Knesset members. The next day I was discharged!

COMING HOME!

Two weeks were up and I reminded both the physiotherapy fellow and the nurse about this anticipated day the day before. It seemed they needed the reminder. I also stressed that my son would be coming to pick me up at a precise hour and that I want to be sure to leave on time since he's a very busy guy with six children. The nurse gave me the envelope packed with papers on time! No word of instruction. Later I wish she'd said something in particular. I didn't bother calling the hospital afterwards.

The woman who represents the home care company came around to us in the hospital to sign us up for a caregiver. This is essential. She was Arabic-speaking. It was a bit confusing since there was also a social worker at the Assuta hospital who had introduced herself to me. Anyway, I agreed to a caregiver right away and happy I did so. Michael had enough clients of his own and works long hours and does a lot of bussing to each one. The young Arabic-speaking caregiver and I hit it off right away. We even now feel friendship between us. After a while when I felt better she taught me how to make the Arabic dish called, Maqluba. She made way too much so I took some over to one of our son's families (five people). Maybe one day I'll surprise someone and make it. I'm not a real cook; my husband is. We're blessed and eat well. Someone wrote a book, *You Are What You Eat*. I haven't read it, but I agree. I'm especially concerned for children who don't have a proper breakfast. I think some are in a bad mood at school and not learning properly because of this. It makes me sad. When my children were growing up we didn't have much money and if you ask them they'll tell you about the three or four types of hot cereal I made for them in the mornings. They learned well since they all have a degree in higher education PTL! I made sure they drank enough water as well.

The woman, mentioned above, representing the caregivers was "beating the system." She was concerned that no time be lost. The system demands that the home care is "cleared" by the National Insurance. The National Insurance (in Hebrew Bituah Leumi) is slow about getting things done. She came the day or two after I was home and helped me fill out the forms and get things rolling. When it came to physiotherapy I was in a daze.

I told you that I received the envelope of many papers. If the nurse had told me simply, "You're on your own now to make appointments for PT, I would have understood. Maybe I thought they would do this for us. They did more than enough, believe me. My caregiver, who also knew Hebrew and English got on the phone to PT on her first visit to me. I thought she was smart and courageous. A few days passed and I was getting nervous but eventually the "home" physiotherapist showed up. My feet were very swollen at the ankles since I was no longer bandaging them as they had done at the hospital.

The surgeon had told me to come with x-ray in hand after six weeks. I made an appointment after one month, however. He said I was doing fine but to bandage the legs from the ankle up (as we'd done at the hospital). I did this and it was only a matter of time until the swelling had gone down. Weeks after I was home I received a call from the National Insurance. They offered me laundry service at no cost and adult diapers. Thankfully I didn't need these! I also need to mention that they sent a person to check on the caregiver. They made clear that window cleaning was not included in the jobs a caregiver was supposed to do. I assured them that I was satisfied with what she had done so far for me. I couldn't clean my own floors and she could do them well. She washed dishes a couple of times. I did have her do a few things which were "off limits" but she did them without making a fuss. The time came when I realized the only thing I really needed from her was to take me to appointments in her car. She did this and it was greatly appreciated. Not every caregiver has a car so I felt this was a great blessing from the Lord.

Somehow I got a person from National Insurance on the phone who told me that if I no longer needed the caregiver, but was still eligible for one, I could get money instead. This was wonderful news. I felt the Lord was involved here since two different payments came through when I needed them. The caregiver herself decided she wanted to take on a different type of work and I needed to officially "free her" from her company, which I did. I hope someone in my situation who feels that they no longer need help, will make sure they get the money which they deserve to get.

Back to the physiotherapist. He came to my home once or twice a week and the workouts were excellent. It's important to keep moving. He taught me how to go up and down steps and I do pretty well on them. I wrote down all of the exercises each time and tried my best to follow through daily.

MONTHS AFTER SURGERY

During my recovery time I developed a terrible tooth ache and once my son helped, and another time the caregiver drove me at a distance for a dental appointment. The end of the story is pending. The pain from it was WORSE than the knee operation! For a couple of days I felt useless. I just lay in bed and didn't even read a book. Since we're on the subject of teeth, I'll take a big loop before I "get back on the highway." My serious operations were covered by my insurance. Why shouldn't they be? I worked in Israel for 33 years and was part of a system! Dental work wherever you go in the world is expensive. Lately I understood that the best solution for the affected tooth is extraction and an implant. I mention my husband's and my trip to Italy later in the book. The price for the dental work is equal to what we spent on that amazing trip abroad! Please folks, take care especially of the children's teeth. I made a mistake as a mother one summer when I purchased a juice concentrate which was tasty, but which caused us terrible dental bills. After this we switched to water. Sweet drinks are great for parties, otherwise you may be sorry. I also recommend sweets only on the weekends. Just grandmother talk… sorry!

I had asked the doctor at the Italian hospital when I could swim. She said six weeks. I went back in the seventh week and started slowly. Don't forget to "freeze" your account if you're a member of a sport facility and won't be there for a long time! It wasn't long before I began doing physiotherapy at the clinic to which I would have to travel by bus. There when I was supposed to work on the exercise bike, I FROZE. I was afraid to make the pedal go around even once. The trainer couldn't force me. I didn't want to disappoint him, however. I went to the pool a couple times after this and determined to do the frog kick while swimming on my back. This stroke required lots of knee bends. In another week when I needed to ride the exercise bike, I was able to pedal for five minutes. Hooray! And the next time ten minutes. It's far easier to exercise in the water. I continue to swim doing this stroke every other time together with the crawl. So then, why, if I'm doing this and walking twice a day on my "off" days, do I need a pain pill? I take an Optalgin sometimes once a day. I'm not using ice any more on the knees like I was doing in the earlier months. I guess I'm getting better after all.

The home physiotherapy person recommended that I see a specialist in his department for lymph since I had swelling. Can you believe how long I had to wait for her? September 20th (keeping in mind my surgery was end of May). When the day finally came, the appointment with the lymph lady was cancelled. I rescheduled but then she cancelled again and again. When I finally got to see her she could see I was upset. This simply doesn't happen in the Maccabi system. She abruptly asked me who referred me to her. I told her. She left the room. After a little while she explained that she didn't recommend a cuff for the knee since it would prevent the "bend." She gave me a few exercises which I'm doing. At the end of the visit, noting that I didn't look "Israeli" she asked what brought me to Israel. Dear reader, if you don't know Israelis, be prepared – we have the word "hutzpa" which means "nerve." I was up to the challenge and told her I was like Ruth. "Which Ruth?" Ruth in the Bible, I replied. She married Boaz. Now she understood. I decided to spill it all out. I told her we were Messianics. My husband is Jewish but there's no conflict since we believe in the same "Yeshua." She said that she had worked for an old folks' home in the German Colony. I offered, "The Ebenezer Home." She said, "Yes, that's it." I told her it's the ONLY home in Israel for Messianic believers. "Weren't you aware about our faith?" I told her not to be afraid to read the New Testament. She replied, "I'm not afraid of ANYTHING!" Wow. I invited her to our congregation which is next to that home and said there's a program for her daughters. (I had seen them on a previous occasion). This was a Divine Appointment and now I see why it was being blocked. She has something to think about. She had taught physiotherapy at Ebenezer Home years ago in place of a woman, whom she named, who was on maternity leave. By the time I saw her, the swelling in my knee had subsided; nevertheless, I believe her exercises are worth doing and I do them.

When I scheduled the appointment with the surgeon the first time, it was two weeks before he had said to come. I didn't bring the x-ray. I already mentioned that he gave me the key for bringing the swelling down. The next appointment would be in September, after another three months. I was a bit discouraged. I was taking medicines daily in June like Optalgin, Acamol, and Ibuphen. When I told him this, he recommended not to take Ibuphen if possible since it's hard on the liver. From that point on I tried to do without it. I would take it if I was going somewhere, for example. He simply reminded me that the healing can take from six months to one year. Encouraging or discouraging? You decide. I can't complain. I get around for shopping and attend events. I even traveled on the train to a musical in English, close to Jerusalem. My daughter met up with me there. A night out! But, woe is me; I forgot evidence of the vaccines (the GREEN passport!). We already arrived late. Thank G-d for the younger generation. She got to a site on her IPhone which confirmed me as "green" and we went inside. We were unable to get to our wonderful seats in the 6th row. Most of words in that first part evaded me (hopefully I'll get ahold of the DVD of it and watch it). After the break we got to our seats and I could hear much better. My legs were sore at night but it was worth it. Then just two weeks ago I traveled to Jerusalem to participate in a choir concert. I took Ibuphen as a precaution. Again, the leg bothers me but I can't say I'm in severe pain.

Assuta Hospital wanted to know what we thought of their services. They had a follow-up questionnaire and the link showed up on my simple cell phone as well as in my email box. They provided it in English as well as Hebrew. I would fill in my identity number and year of birth and that's as far as it went. This went on about six times. I would write back and tell them there was a problem. FINALLY, six months after surgery it worked. They were great as a hospital but apparently don't have the best computer expert. I gave them praise. Yes, I've basically returned to my pre-surgery activities. No, I'm not depressed, PTL!

THOSE "CONTROVERSIAL" MINISTRIES

There are folks which believe in the five-fold ministries. We have them listed in Ephesians 4:11 "So Christ himself gave the apostles, the prophets, the evangelists, the pastors and teachers." All evangelicals believe in this book of Ephesians written by Paul and teach it. Some have a problem with apostles and prophets, however. They aren't sure who the modern-day apostles are. They don't know if the prophets ceased to be after Bible times. Lately, particularly in 2020, there were many prophets, I suppose mostly in the U.S.A. who were prophesying in regards to the election outcome. Things didn't come out the way they prophesied. There was growing mistrust in their so-called biblical authority and doubts remain in many people's minds to this day.

Two famous people with healing ministries visited Israel years ago. Benny Hinn had a meeting at the Sea of Galilee Amphitheater and it was packed. I was very impressed with the meeting and although some people find fault with him, at that particular time I thought everything which occurred in that meeting was fine. Then Maurice Cerullo came to Jerusalem. Believers in the land were invited to stay in a nice hotel for three or four days for free and to attend the meetings. I took the children out of school for those days and it was a blessed experience. The children listened attentively; there was no program specifically for them. They had to listen in English, not their native tongue. There was nice music. The goal of the conference was not only for those who needed healing to be healed, but to be empowered for others. On the last night he invited us to come forward. He held a big bowl of oil in his hands and came to each one of us and touched our foreheads with the oil and prayed for us. I have a little bottle of anointing oil and have used it when praying for people.

Maurice came back years later and held an evening meeting in Tel Aviv. I drove there with a friend from Scandinavia. There was a lot of road work going on and we sadly wandered around too long and missed most of the meeting. We did hear some good words from him and went forward at the end. The huge camera was recording what was going on. In Israel usually the congregations don't allow visitors to photograph them or to take videos. We had no choice. It was a very big crowd. Sid Roth was a guest in the Russian-speaking congregation of Daniel Mattias years ago. The subject there was the occult. People came forward who had been involved with this and were prayed for and delivered. I don't remember if there were any healings at that time but he is known well for his ministry of healing, via television and internet. I read Kathryn Kuhlman's book, *I Believe in Miracles*, and didn't have any problem with it.

MORE POST-SURGERY MUSINGS

I wrote notes about people I met and conversations I had with them while in the hospital, including the nurses. I won't include this information in this book but I know I had some "Divine appointments" for sharing and praying. I was impressed with two employees there in particular. They happened to be Arabic-speaking Muslims. I felt that the Lord wanted me to give them a gift long after I would be back home and recovered and able to walk in without a cane. I prayed that when I came they would be there and that no one else would see that I'm giving them something (so they would wonder or be jealous). I finally arrived and gave the gifts to those two people with no problem at all (G-d answered that specific prayer). In one case it was a lovely Bible in Arabic since he had truly shown interest when I told him about Yeshua. I also had a thank you plaque ready to present to the nurses. There are many hanging on the walls. They really liked it. It even had my picture on it to remind them of who I am.

Have you seen the pattern of my journey through life? Sometimes I relied on the nurses and doctors. At other times I received Yeshua's healing. I believe in the case of the healings that they were genuine. I don't regret any of them and I've shared the incidents with others throughout my lifetime. I think we can see that even if a healing meant delaying the surgery, it was valid. I believe G-d has given to us the know-how; namely, those gadgets which are inserted in the body to enable us to walk for more years on this earth without pain. If someone wants to believe that our miracle G-d can even cause those original bones to grow in place and replace the "robot" material, they can be my guest. I have yet to meet this person with their x-rays in hand, however, I'm open to it.

What about miraculous healings today? I feel that in many cases the reason why there are supernatural healings in the third world countries is because they lack the hospital and medical personnel to perform the needed operations on the people. G-d is a merciful, compassionate G-d. There are stories of miraculous healings in the USA this year; 2021. I believe any report but am cautious for reasons which I've stated above. As for Israel, if G-d's power is being poured out and someone has been healed recently, I'd truly be rejoicing. Generally I believe the Body here needs to awaken to Holy Spirit power. I've been here for many years and I have yet to come across a fellowship in which people are truly praying for revival and for the supernatural gifts to be evident, as compared with the Mount Zion Fellowship. And speaking of them, I need to mention that it was connected with the Ashland, Virginia campground where year after year people would come, even long-term and hear these teachings and experience healing. Recently I read the book by the successor to Ruth Heflin, named Jane Lowder. She and Harold McDougal wrote *A Foretaste of Glory Divine.* She tells us about miracle healings which took place in various countries of the world which she visited. She saw the blind see and the lame walk. My review of her book appears on the amazon site. She is pastor and director of Calvary Campground. One can even find her videos online.

Since I'm trying to recall as many health-related incidents as possible, here is more. I had mentioned my hearing aids. 2021 was my "renewal year." I updated my glasses. I needed only a small change of number. It was mostly for "vanity" reasons; to appear in a newer style of glasses. The last job I had before going onto pension was at an accounting firm. I was there for more than ten years as the "mother tongue" English typist. I needed to type thousands and thousands of numbers during that time into many, many charts. We prepared annual reports for many of the multi-million dollar companies in the world. The Lord protected my eyes during that time. In addition, I've always been an avid reader and continue to read a book every week or two. I have 144 reviews of books on amazon as of now. Could it be that my regular practice of weekly fasting helped my eyes? I believe it did. I knew for years that my hearing wasn't good and I finally went for testing just before the corona lockdowns. Since I wasn't out and about, I didn't need to do anything. When we came out of the lockdown I was fortunate that I didn't need to do the testing again. I simply went and ordered my aids not too far from my home. They were subsidized by my medical plan and were very reasonable. I'm so grateful to the Lord for the technology the Lord has given to us. I had been in healing meetings in which the leader would tell us that some folks' hearing was being restored. I was not in that category. Both eye glasses and hearing aids are essential for us if we're not healed. These impairments are not a disease. Any contact with those involved, whether it is doctors, examiners, or marketing folks, present opportunities to share Yeshua. I live in a comfort zone. I don't mind being alone most of the time. At my age I don't feel the need for a social life apart from attending the congregation. I have accumulated many "acquaintances," particularly via the modern media, but as for a circle of true friends, if I can't count them on the fingers of one hand it doesn't disturb me. I have a prayer partner of many, many years. She would be considered my best friend but during covid-19 we were praying via Skype on the computer. I don't know why I'm sharing this. I don't speak much about my beliefs and the contents of this book. I feel that if a person is seeking more of Yeshua, He will reveal Himself to them and make everything clear to them. When we're yielded to Him life becomes very simple. I feel that many folks waste lots of time with things which aren't worthwhile and I'm sad about this. Do I mean we should all become bookworms? Well, to a certain degree, yes. Old folks, no longer working who aren't reading would be a wonderment for me. I wonder what they're doing with their time.

Once when I was working at the accounting firm, I needed to work from the morning, all night until the morning. They ordered a special taxi for me to arrive home in Migdal HaEmek, about 35 km. away. I walked in and greeted my family with "Good morning!" I developed sciatic nerve pain for many weeks as a result of sitting so many hours. I bought a special "back" to put on my chair called Dr. Gav ("gav" is the Hebrew word for back) and would carry it to work and back to ease the back pain. I was offered physiotherapy but didn't go since I had my alternative chiropractor, mentioned before. On another occasion, when I finally went to PT, they applied ultrasound a couple of times and I was fine.

On an occasion years later, when I went for a checkup to Maccabi, the physiotherapist recommended joining group therapy for the back. We met six times and it was helpful. I fully realize the importance of doing a round of exercises every day, in addition to walking or swimming. It takes discipline and I don't get around to them as often as I know I should.

Within the year before covid-19 I moved incorrectly and needed to go for back treatments. I started a series of appointments with the alternative chiropractor via my Maccabi health plan. He did "hands on" treatments and it was helpful. I told him about my knee problems and the last couple of visits out of eight visits he worked on the knees. He told me that my legs were uneven, even by as much as four centimeters. After treatments the gap had lessened to less than two centimeters. Even now after the knee surgery my legs are uneven.

I recommend the alternative methods. Years ago I went to an alternative woman, who, together with her husband, took the "points" of the hands and feet. A believer had recommended this Clinica Laniado. I traveled a great distance to them. It meant a change of diet. I complied, eating orange things, like lentils, and also salmon, and basmati rice. I didn't eat tomatoes and cucumbers for a while. Something happens with the body pH. I also took three types of "homeopathic" drops which were from the USA and very expensive. I felt better afterwards. I told our believing doctor in Haifa about this and he mentioned that those drops could be dangerous for the liver. He also told me that the car

I was driving was bad for my back. He recommended swimming. It could be that upon that advice I began my year-around swimming which I'm sure was a great key to avoiding further circulation and back problems.

At one point in my life a doctor told me that due to cholesterol, I could eat beef only at a special event once in a given year. Do you think I believed him? Also once the thyroid was an issue. I DID have it checked recently at my daughter's suggestion but it's not far enough out of range to worry about.

Aren't you glad that G-d gave us three basic things to keep in mind in order to be healthy; namely, good sleep, good, healthy food and exercise. As for sleep, I think many people walk around sleep-deprived. My father lived to be 99. He was good at "self-mastery." When he was hungry he ate, and when he was tired, he slept. I am like him in this regard. I told my daughter when she was in high school to go to bed no later than 10 p.m. if she wanted to remain beautiful. Now she's a mother of two small tots and I'm happy to report that since she needs to get up very early to drop them off, and then go to work, she makes it a point to get to bed early. When a person is sleep-deprived they tend to be cranky. The world doesn't need cranks!

As for diet, cooking healthy, natural foods is the best policy, as opposed to "prepared" foods. Exercise is necessary especially for those of us who are pensioners and no longer having to walk around or to a work place. I had mostly sit-down jobs, but one also walks more, like to the car and back. Seniors need to walk around the block a few times if they're not members of some sport center. Stationary bikes are good, if one can afford them. Also, if you know a round of exercises you can do in your living room, just do them! Do you know about the "leaning camel" or "scared cat" exercises (on all fours) for the lower back? They're easy to do and very helpful.

Do we know the importance of making valuable use of time even when we're suffering? When I wrote my last two books for sale on amazon (about Capernwray), not only was it during lockdown, but I also had a bout with shingles. I could never have made it without the help of my husband. It required daily showers and medicine to be applied on oozing sores. Most of the sores were on the back. It was painful but I continued to type and type at my computer until my hands would even be sore at the end of the day.

TAKE TIME

Here's something about time:

Take time to think. It is the source of power. Take time to play. It is the doorway to perpetual youth.

Take time to read. It is the foundation of wisdom. Take time to pray. It is the greatest power on earth.

Take time to be friendly. It is the road to happiness. Take time to laugh. It is the music of the soul.

Take time to give. The day is too short to be selfish. We have no time to lose. Let's use it for the things that are worthwhile.

Just for Today – Lord for tomorrow & its needs I do not pray; Keep me my God from stain of sin,

Just for today.

Now set a seal upon my lips, For this I pray; Keep me from wrong or idle words,

Just for today.

Let me be slow to do my will, Prompt to obey, And keep me, guide me, use me Lord,

Just for today.

* *

A lot of believers are like wheelbarrows – not good unless pushed.

Some are like canoes – they need to be paddled.

Some are like kites – if you don't keep a string on them, they fly away.

Some are like footballs – you can't tell which way they will bounce next.

Some are like balloons – full of wind and ready to blow up.

Some are like trailers – they have to be pulled.

Some are like neon lights – they keep going on and off.

Some are like a good watch – open face, pure gold, quietly busy and full of good works.

(Slovak Courier)

* *

Do more than exist, live. Do more than touch, feel. Do more than look, observe.

Do more than hear, listen. Do more than listen, understand. Do more than think, ponder.

Do more than talk, say something.

WORLDWIDE PANDEMIC

The corona period was difficult for the entire world. Millions died. If you lost a loved one or friend, I sorrow and weep with you. At the same time, I honestly feel it was a spiritual wake-up call to the world to repent and be ready to meet the one true G-d. Many have been saved through this period. One thing I know is that G-d will not remove anyone from this earth one hour sooner or later than was intended from before they were born. Psalm 139:16 “Your eyes saw my substance, being yet unformed. And in Your book they all were written, The days fashioned for me, When as yet there were none of them.”

The true believer has assurance of eternal life. I don’t believe in “once saved always saved.” I believe we have to walk the walk and talk the talk. Better to be a true follower of Yeshua, than to be half-way and then be surprised when we stand face to face with Him. I'm looking forward to my heavenly home. I'm looking forward to my new, glorified body like Yeshua had after His resurrection from the dead. After speaking with Yeshua in "Gan Eden" (the Hebrew concept of eternity is the original Garden of Eden), I'm looking forward to meeting the great Bible heroes, the martyrs and the notable saints who have gone before. We'll even automatically know about their ministries; the thousands who found faith through them and the thousands who were healed through their ministries. How about this thought?

FAITH HEALERS IN ISRAEL

I have mentioned that Benny Hinn and Maurice Cerullo had been in Israel. Their meetings were not announced in the congregations, unless perhaps at Kehilat HaCarmel in Haifa. As of this writing most of the congregations don't believe in the Baptism of the Holy Spirit, as described by these historical preachers listed in the chapter below.

The Israeli ministry Revive Israel/Global Tikkun states on their website that they, quote: are actively committed to all the work and fruit and charismatic gifts of the Holy Spirit (I Corinthians 12) in our lives, being sensitive to the leading of the Spirit in everything we say and do. Unquote. They would be the closest to agreeing with this book. I attended their all-night prayer meeting on the grounds of Yad HaShmona during Shavuot years ago. The reason was that I lacked transportation to arrive at the believer's picnic the following day at that location. I didn't find it easy to stay up all those hours. I prefer to fast for days than lose sleep. During the day time I was walking through David's Citadel and sprained my ankle, not seeing a step. I was in pain. A young woman attending this prayer meeting prayed for my ankle and I felt instant relief. I do believe the Lord used her as a conduit of healing.

In 1994 my husband completed the Associate degree in Bible/Theology at the Galilee Bible College of the Assemblies of God in Haifa. This course is no longer offered. The students were Russian or Arabic-speaking. At the end of the course the students were offered a position in that denomination. If I'm not mistaken, none of the Russian-speakers agreed, however, part of the Arabic speakers became a part. Ross Beyer was principal and Sam Brelo was the dean.

I had three divine healings at the feast of tabernacles. The first was via Martie Haaijer, the second via Christine Darg and the third via Paul O'Higgins. All of them have written books. I don't know how one can get ahold of Martie Haaijer's book. Paul prayed for my LEFT knee. It wasn't healed for about four years until I lost five kilos. Do you realize how our weight can deter us? A simple lifestyle of prayer and fasting might be the key for many people. In my background we never fasted. Fasting was something the Pentecostals (Mt. Zion Fellowship) practiced in Jerusalem. We fasted TOO OFTEN in my humble opinion but we survived.

In the early 1990's when our family first began attending the feast there were two different people offering healing meetings in the morning. Mahesh Chavda was one of them. He and his wife have many books for sale. Andrew White, the Vicar of Baghdad, Iraq, a previous feast speaker has a book for sale which includes healing miracles. Gwen Shaw, founder of End-Time Handmaidens, went to Shanghai, China as a missionary when she was 23. She ministered in various countries of the world and healing was a part of her ministry. She was a feast speaker and also wrote books. There is an extensive book list on her website of spiritual books for believers. She passed away in 2013. Charlotte Baker (Dr.) pastored King's Temple for 18 years in Seattle, Washington. She also helped established a Bible college in Ghana. She retired in Canada and died in 2014 at the age of 92. She has written books, including one of a prophecy which she received. She believed in the ministry gifts. Her husband was not a preacher but he supported her. She was a memorable feast speaker.

I remember the first year Apostle Rene Terra Nov arrived to speak at the evening service of the feast. This was when the Dutch founders , Johann Luckhoff (Dr.) and Jan Willem van der Hoeven were the leaders. Johann Luckhoff was unsure if Rene would arrive on time all the way from Manaus, Brazil. Since that time he has spoken in seminars, as a speaker the opening night at Ein Gedi and in the evening meetings. He is the founder and Senior Apostle of Ministerio Internacional da Restaurcion (MIR) in Manaus. With his wife Apostle Ana Marita, the church grew from 100 people to over seventy thousand using the model of cell churches. Apostle Terra Nova develops leaders throughout Brazil and other nations to now include over seven million members worldwide. The network is the 4th largest Pentecostal-Charismatic network in the world - and continues to grow. Healing and tongues is part of the ministry.

Pastor Sandor Nemeth, of the Faith Church of Budapest, Hungary, was a featured speaker at the Feast of Tabernacles. This church is part of the Pentecostal/Charismatic movement. On the website it states that they believe in the gifts of the Holy Spirit, including healing. He pastors the largest growing church in the European Union. There are 70,000 active members and 300 local groups, both around Hungary and abroad.

William (Billy) Wilson is the President of Oral Roberts University in Tulsa, Oklahoma. In 2006, Wilson served as the executive officer for the Azusa Street Centennial in Los Angeles, California. This revival drew more than 50,000 people from 106 nations. He was a feast speaker. He has written books, including one on the importance of fasting.

Dr. Paul Enenche is a trained medical doctor but who has also held huge healing meetings. Located in Abuja, Nigeria, they have TV broadcasts, internet and mass media productions which reach millions. They began small in 1996 and now have tens of thousands of members. The church auditorium was completed in the year 2018 and made the landmark of 100,000 seating capacity to be regarded as the largest church auditorium in the world as of then. He was the featured speaker the first night of the feast at Ein Gedi in 2014.

Reinhard Bonnke spoke at the opening night of the feast at the Dead Sea in 2017. He was the "Billy Graham of Africa." He has been said to have 77 million recorded conversions to Jesus Christ through his crusades. A book which records many miracles is called *Living a Life of Fire*.

Daniel Kolenda is a modern missionary evangelist who has led more than 21 million people to Christ through massive open air evangelistic campaigns in some of the most dangerous difficult and remote locations on earth. He is the successor of world renowned Reinhard Bonnke. He spoke at the ICEJ opening Ein Gedi celebration in 2018. Attended by thousands of people from all over the world, he shared the story of his grandfather who was born with an abnormally-sized head. He was on his deathbed. People had gathered for the funeral but the boy's father stayed in prayer in a nearby room. He would come out from time to time, telling the folks that G-d was working.

In the perfect time, G-d healed the boy. He became the father of ten sons. There are many preachers in that family. Daniel is the president and CEO of Christ for All Nations. Their students believe in teaching, preaching and healing. At the end of the service in Ein Gedi many people went forward for healing, salvation or rededication. One can purchase this message on ICEJ's website (bookstore).

19th-20th Century
FAITH HEALERS

1843-1919 **A.B. Simpson** was a Canadian preacher, theologian, author, and founder of the Christian and Missionary Alliance (C&MA) - an evangelical denomination with an emphasis on global evangelism.

The young Albert was raised in a strict Calvinistic, Scottish Presbyterian and Puritan tradition. A visiting evangelist from Ireland made a strong impression on him during a revival in 1859. He went to college and university and became a minister in a Presbyterian church. By the age of 21, he was already pastoring a very large church in Ontario, Canada.

He later moved to Kentucky, in the USA, to pastor a large church. Afterwards, he moved to New York City, but resigned as a pastor to work among the new immigrants and many poor communities of New York.

He published the first missionary journal in 1882, called "The Gospel in All Lands." He also published a color magazine which became the official publication of the missionary organization he founded.

Simpson began teaching ministers and missionaries, to prepare them for multi-cultural situations. His school was eventually called the Nyack Collage and Alliance Theological Seminary. He was known as a very effective communicator of the Word of God. Once he was miraculously healed of a lifelong illness, and this became part of his teaching as well. He would devote one meeting a week for teaching, testimonies and prayer for healing. Other churches did not accept this.

The organization which he began was non-denominational. He outlined the plan for the way a Christian church should be a home for the needy, as well as an armory where the believers would be equipped to fight spiritual battles in a sinful world.

Simpson composed the lyrics of over 120 hymns. Many of the Assemblies of God and Church of the Foursquare Gospel had leaders who had received their training at Nyack College. There are churches in Peru, Philippines and India which bear his name.

Nearly 100 years have passed since Simpson's death, but the chorus of one of his songs remains in the minds of many believers today; namely, "Yesterday, Today, Forever, Jesus is the Same."

1844-1924 Maria Woodworth-Etter was an American healing evangelist. Her ministry style would serve as a model for Pentecostalism.

Woodworth-Etter was born again at the age of 13. She felt the call to bring others to know the Lord. She was married and had six children, but five of them died at a young age. She divorced her husband due to infidelity and later remarried.

She read the Scriptures and began to preach the Lord's divine will in healing. Many were won to Christ as a result of seeing others healed. She pioneered the way for Pentecostal manifestations that are so common among Charismatic and Pentecostal groups today.

She attended a Disciples of Christ congregation, but they did not allow women to preach. She found support in a local Quaker meeting. She received the baptism of the Holy Spirit and began to hold meetings. Hundreds of people came to hear her and reporters from across the country wrote articles about the meetings. For a while she was a part of the Church of God.

She began to pray for the sick in 1885, believing that those with sufficient faith would be healed. Sometimes people would fall to the floor during her meetings and later tell others about their experiences. She eventually purchased a tent which held 8,000 people. In 1912, she joined the young Pentecostal movement and preached widely in Pentecostal circles until her death, helping found the Assemblies of God in 1914.

In 1918, she founded what is today Lakeview Church (Temple) of Indianapolis, Indiana.

1854-1930 Alexander Boddy was an Anglican vicar and one of the founders of Pentecostalism in Britain.

Boddy was born into an ecclesiastical family: his father was a vicar, and his mother was a descendant of Mary Vazeille, who had been married to John Wesley. Although he trained to be a solicitor, a religious experience at the Keswick Convention convinced him he should become ordained into the Church of England.

During this time in Britain, very few were praying for outpourings of the Holy Spirit. As a result, the movement reached the USA, India, Germany, Holland and Scandinavia first. The reaction of most Christians in Britain at the time was unfavorable.

Boddy loved to travel and kept diaries. Once, he managed to travel to Russia, where the Russian Tsar saw his book and made him a member of the Imperial Geographical Society of Russia. He wrote about Barbary and was also made a fellow of their geographical society. After visiting Israel, he wrote *Days of Galilee*.

Boddy was inspired by the Holiness Movement, and in 1892, he had an intense religious experience. In 1899, his wife Mary experienced a healing from asthma and they both believed that she had a gift for healing through the laying-on of hands. In 1904, he visited Wales during the Welsh Revival and met Evan Roberts. The following year he travelled to Oslo, where

T. B. Barratt was leading a religious revival modelled on the events of the Azusa Street Revival in Los Angeles. Barratt was invited to Boddy's church, and subsequently Boddy and his wife began to experience speaking in tongues. Smith Wigglesworth visited and the Boddy's laid hands on him. The Sunderland Conventions gained national press attention. The Whitsun conventions went on for seven years until WW I broke out. Pentecostal leaders from many parts of the world came to speak, as well as some outstanding Lutheran pastors from Germany. Reporters were not allowed. Sometimes one or two would begin to sing during the prayer. Others would then join and it was like a heavenly choir, being joined by angels. The music was without words.

Although Boddy was active in Pentecostal organizations, since he was a Church of England minister, he was against separate denominations. He began the first Pentecostal publication in Britain, called "Confidence." He taught that divine love was more important than speaking in tongues. He was cautious about healing testimonies. When visiting the USA, he was disturbed to see the emphasis on money among the Pentecostal churches. Unlike some other Pentecostals, he supported the British war effort.

1859-1947 Smith Wigglesworth was a British evangelist who was influential in the early history of Pentecostalism.

Wigglesworth was born into a poor family and when very young had to work in the fields, pulling turnips together with his mother. He also worked in factories in order to help provide the family. He was illiterate.

He became born again at eight years old. His family was Methodist, but they also attended Anglican churches. He learned the trade of plumbing from a man in the Brethren movement.

He married a woman who was a preacher with the Salvation Army. They had five children together, before she passed away at age 31. She had taught him to read the Bible after they were married. It was the only book he ever read. He did not permit newspapers in their home. Eventually he left plumbing and began preaching. He had a "laying-on of hands" experience through a revivalist, resulting in speaking in tongues. He spoke at some of the Assemblies of God events in Great Britain. He also received ministerial credentials with the Assemblies of God in the United States, where he evangelized during the 1920s and later.

Wigglesworth believed that healing came through faith, and he was flexible in his approach. Once, when he was forbidden to lay hands on audience members, by the authorities in Sweden, he preached for a "corporate healing", by which people laid hands on themselves. He also practiced anointing with oil, and the distribution of "prayer handkerchiefs" (one of which was sent to King George V). Wigglesworth sometimes attributed ill-health to demons.

Smith largely believed his ministerial success was due to his speaking in tongues. He said:

"I want you to see that he that speaketh in an unknown tongue edifieth himself or builds himself up. We must be edified before we can edify the church. I cannot estimate what I, personally, owe to the Holy Ghost method of spiritual edification. I am here before you as one of the biggest conundrums in the world. There never was a weaker man on the platform. Language? None. Inability–full of it. All natural things in my life point exactly opposite to my being able to stand on the platform and preach the gospel. The secret is that the Holy Ghost came and brought this wonderful edification of the Spirit. I had been reading this Word continually as well as I could, but the Holy Ghost came and took hold of it, for the Holy Ghost is the breath of it, and He illuminated it to me."

Wigglesworth spoke in many countries throughout the world. His sermons appeared in Pentecostal magazines and were later collected into two books: *Ever Increasing Faith* and *Faith that Prevails*. There are accounts of various healings which occurred during his ministry, including resurrections from the dead.

1862-1940 Thomas Ball Barratt was a British-born Norwegian pastor and one of the founding figures of the Pentecostal movement in Europe, bringing the movement, or baptism in the Holy Spirit, as it became known, to Norway and Europe in 1906. He was originally a

Methodist pastor but later left the church and went on to establish the Pentecostal movement in Norway.

He was involved in charitable work and also fought against alcohol. He was a sought-after preacher and wrote several books and a number of theological articles in Christian publications.

Barratt was fluent in English and Norwegian from a very young age. He attended a Methodist school in England and received salvation at age 12. He attended Wesleyan Collegiate Institute, now known as Queen's College in Taunton, Somerset, England, and also studied art and music. He also studied under composer Edvard Grieg in Norway.

Barratt began preaching at age 17 and pastored in several Methodist churches in Norway. He wrote articles for Christian publications. He traveled to New York to raise money in order to enlarge his church building. He rented a room in preacher A.B.Simpson's guesthouse in Manhattan. This house became part of the Christian and Missionary Alliance. He did not succeed in his money-raising. While there he heard about the Azusa Street Revival in Los Angeles. He had wanted to be baptized in the Holy Spirit. He came across one of their newsletters and wrote a letter to them. The reply he received changed his life. He had his breakthrough in 1906 and was baptized in the Holy Spirit. The following month he experienced another breakthrough as he spoke and sang in tongues.

He felt like the prophet Daniel, when he had encountered the supernatural, and slid onto the floor. He had a supernatural experience seeing fire, and others saw at the same time a strong red light. He began to speak in a foreign language. Early in the morning he continued to speak in tongues in several languages. He also sang in the Spirit and his voice became clear and strong. He wrote to Norway about this experience. People in Los Angeles had experienced awakening and he felt he was the first in New York to have experienced a similar visitation of G-d.

Barratt returned to Norway in December 1906 without funds or church support. With his return, his baptism in the Spirit caused a stir. Revival broke out in Oslo upon his return. Once when he desired to tell the congregation about his baptism in the Spirit he could only stand there crying. He left the podium without having preached. Shortly afterwards a Pentecostal revival after Christmas took place and continued all night. By the New Year ten people had been baptized in the Spirit in Oslo. This marked the start of the Pentecostal movement in Norway.

He was no longer connected with the Methodist churches. He would preach in various churches or rent buildings. He split from others and his movement became the Norwegian Pentecostal movement. A Pentecostal assembly which he began in Oslo, continues to this day.

Many Christians in Norway considered these people to be fanatics. When he went for walks rotten eggs were thrown at him. The revival in Oslo spread, however. The movement attracted international attention. Some came from other countries to see what was happening and were convinced of its divine origin. They became leaders of the Pentecostal movement in their respective countries. When invited to visit Newcastle in 1907, his preaching marked the beginning of the meeting at All Saints' Church in Sunderland, under the ministry of Boddy. Barratt visited Sweden, Finland, Poland, Estonia, Iceland and Denmark.

In 1908, the first Pentecostal congregation in Norway was founded in Skien by C.M. Seehuus, who also became the congregation's first pastor. Seehuus had broken from the Baptist church in Skien, which he had led.

Women became involved in the ministry. He and his wife were eventually baptized in water. He became a humble leader due to all of the criticism and public ridicule he faced in the first years of his ministry.

He was elected President of the Great European Pentecostal Conference in Stockholm in 1939 by a unanimous vote. He remained the pastor of Filadelfia Oslo until his death in 1940.

When Barratt visited Mosjøen, Norway, in 1933, the hall was packed and a long line of people extended down the street; Barratt's visit made a strong impression. In 1932 Barratt began a choir. He was a prolific songwriter and had a large impact on the music of the Pentecostal movement. It is said that he would sit at the piano and play an improvised musical commentary to conversations and discussions. He often played piano while whistling melodies. He wrote lyrics for over one hundred songs and composed melodies for several of his lyrics. He also translated a number of songs into Norwegian. The first Norwegian Pentecostal movement's songbook contains 110 songs which he had written. Another 130 songs had been translated into Norwegian. Many are widely sung.

Barrett established the "Pentecostal Foreign Mission of Norway." Many missionaries were sent especially to Asia and Africa. Later this organization was dissolved and missionaries were sent by individual congregations. Pentecostal churches have sent a high number of missionaries compared to the number of church members.

Up to 20,000 people are said to have lined the streets for his funeral which took place in 1940. He died at the age of 78.

1870-1935 John G. Lake was a Canadian-American leader in the Pentecostal movement that began in the early 20th century, and is known as a faith healer, missionary, and together with Thomas Hezmalhalch, co-founder of the Apostolic Faith Mission of South Africa.

Lake had 16 siblings, though half of them died young. He had less than ten years of education and no formal theological training. He was ordained into the

Methodist ministry at age 21. He worked as roofer and construction worker in Chicago, before returning to his hometown. He worked in real estate and later became a millionaire in life insurance.

When he chose to leave his successful career to become a preacher, he is said to have walked away from a salary of more than one million dollars per year. Lake played a decisive role in the spread of Pentecostalism in South Africa. Afterwards, he evangelized for 20 years along the west coast of the United States. Lake returned to South Africa years later and became one of the first Pentecostal missionaries to introduce speaking in tongues. Various Zionist Christian sects were established in South Africa at this time. His work was controversial in regard to his use of funds. He was accused of staging miraculous healings in his meetings. After his first wife died in South Africa, he returned to the U.S. and remarried. He started an organization called The Divine Healing Institute and opened what he called "Lake's Divine Healing Rooms." Many were established in other states as well. As of today (2018), there are currently 2,002 Healing Rooms in 58 nations, where Christians are trained in divine healing.

1882-1969 Stanley Howard Frodsham was a British pastor, editor, author and teacher and one of the founding figures of the Pentecostal movement in Europe. He was the editor of the Pentecostal Evangel and the author of 15 books.

Frodsham grew up in a Christian home in England. As a young man he read a history of Hudson Taylor which he found inspirational. He later attended a YMCA in London, where he described a conversion experience. He then travelled to Johannesburg, South Africa where he worked for YMCA for a year in a secretarial role - a work that had just been established there. After this he travelled to Canada in 1906.

On his return from Canada in 1908 Frodsham visited Alexander Boddy in his church in Sunderland, where a series of Pentecostal meetings had been taking place. Frodsham describes receiving the baptism in the Holy Spirit and speaking in tongues. He returned to Bournemouth where he hosted the British-Norwegian Pentecostal pioneer, T. B. Barratt in 1909.

Frodsham began publishing a Pentecostal paper, "Victory," that same year. He became a pastor for the Assemblies of God in 1916, and was elected General Secretary within five years. By 1921 he would also be elected as editor of the Pentecostal Evangel, and all other publications of the Assemblies of God. In 1910, Frodsham returned to Canada where he met and married Alice Rowlands. In 1928, he wrote a history of the Pentecostal movement to date, called *With Signs Following*. In all he wrote 15 books throughout his ministry.

In the 1940s Frodsham became involved in the offshoot Latter Rain Movement which led to controversies among Pentecostals of the period and eventually led to

Frodsham's retirement. A resolution of the Assemblies of God was adopted reinforcing their official disapproval for the movement and a statement to that effect was published in The Pentecostal Evangel after Frodsham's retirement. Owing to his writing and editing, Frodsham was affectionately known as "God's prophet with a pen".

1884-1965, Kelso Reavis Glover was a healing evangelist, Bible teacher, and associate of Aimee Semple McPherson at Angelus Temple.

When Glover was studying at the University of California at Berkeley, he was interested in the baptism of the Holy Spirit. His mother sent him an anointed handkerchief in the mail and through this he was healed. He often used the same method himself. He felt like he was going to have a nervous breakdown from the studies and took six months off. During this time he came across some folks who believed in divine healing. He felt that if he were to preach the gospel, it would be better to study from the teacher Himself. Gradually he left his church and was baptized in the Spirit at the Azusa Street Mission. He began several missions in Central California. It was 1917 when he almost quit. He worked in irrigation projects at this time. He heard the preaching of Aimee Semple McPherson and realized that "Pentecost" was G-d's way.

I stood asking God to make me free; asking Him to bring to pass the word which said: "If the Son make you free you shall be free indeed." And the Spirit of the Lord spoke to me and said, "Why don't you take it?" And as He spoke these words a vision came before me of a chain gang... when the Spirit spoke to me and said, "Why don't you take your liberty," I looked down and saw there were no chains on my feet. Jesus had set me free, but I was still walking in the line. And when I saw my feet had no chains on them, I stepped out of the line. (AE, Feb 1930, p.2)

He decided that the Baptism would not only empower his preaching, but would enable him to 'stand in the testing day.' In 1921 he moved, with his wife to Chicago to pastor. A young, A.C. Valdez, also impacted his ministry. Glover's brother was baptized in the Spirit under Valdez's ministry and they conducted campaigns together, both in Chicago and in Modesto. They ministered in New Zealand as well. Glover preached articulately and with passion. Healing and tongues was part of the ministry.

Glover took over pastoring a church in Australia, which came out of the Sunshine Revival under A.C. Valdez. Valdez had been an evangelist. The church needed some structure which Glover brought in. He was involved in the Victorian Bible Institute and demanded that students "hold the line." He dismissed pre-tribulation premillennialism and refuted the common Pentecostal idea that only those baptized in the Holy Spirit would constitute the raptured Bride of Christ. He taught the importance of the baptism of the Holy Spirit and speaking in tongues for power to preach and to witness.

Glover left Australia in 1927, and began ministering at the Angelus Temple. They had a radio broadcast and Demos Shakarian, was influenced through this broadcast. Glover was asked to pray over the animals on Shakarian's ranch. There was a tuberculosis epidemic in California. They prayed for three hours around the corrals. None of the cattle tested positive to the infection. Glover held campaigns in India and returned to Australia at least once.

Glover died at the age of 82, claiming never to have been sick, never had an operation, and only having seen a doctor when he broke his nose and went for physical checkups. His heritage was substantial, if largely forgotten, by the constituencies that he served. In Australia he is remembered as an impressive but short term bible teacher, whereas his influence as a thinker and theological stabilizing force is largely forgotten. In America, he appears only rarely in the literature, and usually in that by people (such as Raymond Cox) who actually heard him preach. Not one of the 'great names', his influence as a teacher-prophet was probably more substantial than can now be properly assessed.

1884-1964 Lewi Pethrus was a Swedish Pentecostal minister who played a decisive role in the formation and development of the Pentecostal movement in his country. In 1964, he founded the political party the Christian Democrats.

Pethrus held manual jobs from the age of ten, being apprenticed to a shoe factory in 1899. That year, he was baptized in the Baptist church in Vänersborg. After emigrating to Norway in 1900, he became co-pastor of the Arendal Baptist Church in 1902, along with Adolf Mildes. He started speaking in tongues, believed by Pentecostals to be evidence of having received the baptism of the Holy Spirit after a series of meetings in Lillestrand. He claimed that the experience happened to him spontaneously and that he did not understand at the time what was happening to him.

Without formal training, he pastored a church for one year. He later attended the Betel Seminary in Stockholm. This seminary had liberal teaching and didn't teach the divinity of Jesus. He regained his strong faith after meeting Jesus in a vision. He served in the military, and later that year pastored a Baptist church.

Pethrus joined the Pentecostal movement in 1907 after meeting the Norwegian Pentecostal minister Thomas Ball Barratt in Oslo. It was then that the doctrine of the baptism in the Holy Spirit and speaking in tongues became clear to him; he claimed: "From that moment I was part of the Pentecostal Revival".

Pethrus became pastor of the Seventh Baptist Church in Stockholm in 1910 and of the Philadelphia Church in 1911. There were disagreements between the churches in Sweden and they split. He wrote words and music to a gospel song. A Bible School was established and a weekly magazine in 1915 and 1916, respectively. The first missionaries were sent out to Brazil. Many missionaries were afterwards sent to Africa, Latin America and continental Europe. They kept ties with North American Scandinavian Pentecostals as well.

In 1942 a high school was founded and in 1945, a daily newspaper. A credit fund was established in 1952 and a radio station, IBRA Radio (now IBRA Media) in Tangier, Morocco, in 1955. In the same year, the Philadelphia Church hosted the Pentecostal World Conference.

Pethrus resigned from the pastorate in 1958. He continued preaching as an itinerant preacher, and established the Lewi Pethrus Trust for Philanthropic Endeavors. In 1964, he spearheaded the founding of Sweden's Christian Democratic Party. He had moved more into the sphere of politics since the 1940s, after denouncing it wholly during the early years of his ministry. The Christian Democrats were culturally conservative but supported the welfare state. His wife Lydia died in 1966. A year before his own death, he was made a Knight Commander of the Order of Vasa. His last sermon was delivered at the annual Nyhem Week Pentecostal convention in 1974, shortly before his death on 4 September. His autobiography was published in 1976.

1887-1947 Charles S. Price (Dr.) Price 's mother died when the was four. His father remarried and Charles loved and respected this woman. He attended a Methodist school up to age 18. He joined the navy but was discharged after a couple months due to a bad knee. He immigrated from England to Canada. He then moved to Washington state to find work. He was saved in a Free Methodist Mission. He was ordained as a minister in that denomination. This denomination was very liberal so he became a Congregationalist pastor for 12 years. He later moved to California and pastored the First Congregational Church of Lodi. In 1921 one of his members had attended the revival of Aimee Semple McPherson in San Jose. Other members attended and were filled with the Holy Spirit. He attended the meeting in order to gather evidence to teach against this doctrine. Instead, he became convicted of his own emptiness. He was seated on the platform with other pastors and when the altar call was given, he publicly responded. At a subsequent meeting at a Baptist church, he was filled with the Spirit and began to speak with other tongues.

He testified of his experience in his own church and 1,000 members also received this experience. It was a revival and they began evangelistic outreaches. People were healed in his meetings. Denominational leaders criticized what was happening in his church. He left that denomination and began the Lodi Bethel Temple. He began to preach in Oregon and British Columbia. In 1923 he preached to over 250,000 in a three-week period and many were healed. Lorne Fox and his family were healed and began their own evangelistic and healing ministry.

Price held meetings in Calgary, Edmonton, Winnipeg, Toronto, Minneapolis, Duluth, St Louis and Belleville, Illinois. In 1926 Price started publishing the "Golden Grain" periodical, which included many testimonies of healings and miracles. In 1928 Price suffered a blow when his lawyer fled with all his funds. His supporters helped to raise some of the money, but he decided to purchase a tent to hold meetings, so that he no longer had to pay large auditorium expenses. He called it the Kanvas Kathedral. It's reported there were 1000 conversions a day the last 10 days of the Belleville meetings. He continued to travel through the northwest over the next several years. Everywhere he went he saw miraculous healings in his meetings and thousands came to Christ. He counted 35,000 conversions in 1928 alone. The constant traveling put a strain on his marriage. By 1930 he and his wife separated. They eventually divorced in the 1930s.

While many ministries shut down or were severely curtailed during the 1930's, due to the depression, Charles S. Price continued to draw thousands to his meetings. In the late 1930s he ministered in Norway, England, Egypt, Palestine, Turkey, Syria, Lebanon, Italy, as well as continuing to speak throughout the US. He started to refer to himself as Dr. Price, which appears to have been an honorary title rather than an educational one. In 1939 Price estimated that he had traveled over a million miles on evangelistic campaigns since he began in 1922. His schedule was demanding. At meetings where he was the main speaker he would speak two or three times a day and often pray for healing well into the night. During the war years it was increasingly difficult to draw large crowds and Price often spoke in churches and camp meetings. In 1940 between mid-March and mid-August he preached 218 times besides holding 35 healing services, and stayed late hours praying for the sick. He gave several community speeches to groups like the Rotary Club, and did radio addresses, all this while traveling 2700 miles by train and 8500 miles by car. In one day alone he spoke five times in Springfield, Missouri.

Price was not affiliated with a particular denomination and his meetings were often supported by multiple churches within an area. He had a special relationship with the Assembly of God denominational leadership and regularly spoke at their camp meetings and in their churches. He was a prolific writer. He wrote several books including: *And Signs Followed; the Life Story of Charles S. Price, The Potter and the Clay, Spiritual and Physical Health, Made Alive, Two Worlds, The Real Faith, You Can Know God Here and Now, Divine Intervention, and Miracles* besides producing his Golden Grain Magazine from 1926 to 1947. He used radio extensively and often preached from Los Angeles, California when he was not on the road. He also taught at the Southern California Bible College and was often asked to fill in for pastors in the Los Angeles area. In 1945 he felt that the Lord was calling him to spend time at home. The next two years were focused on writing, preaching locally, and in rest and prayer.

1890-1944 Aimee Semple McPherson was a Canadian-American Pentecostal evangelist and media celebrity in the 1920s and 1930s, famous for founding the Foursquare Church. McPherson has been noted as a pioneer in the use of modern media, because she used radio to draw on the growing appeal of popular entertainment in North America and incorporated other forms into her weekly sermons at Angelus Temple.

In her time, she was the most publicized Christian evangelist, surpassing Billy Sunday and her other predecessors. She conducted public faith healing demonstrations before large crowds; testimonies conveyed tens of thousands of people healed. McPherson's articulation of the United States being a nation founded and sustained by divine inspiration continues to be echoed by many pastors still today.

McPherson held large evangelistic meetings in many parts of the USA. After settling in the Los Angeles area, 575,000 people attended her meetings in 1920. People would stand in line for hours to get in. Enrollment grew exceeding 10,000, and "Angelus Temple" was advertised to be the largest single Christian congregation in the world. According to church records, they received 40 million visitors within the first seven years.

McPherson knew about the Salvation Army and encouraged people to give towards the needy, particularly following various natural disasters. During the great depression it is said that she fed 1.5 million people. People who had nothing to do with her "Angelus Temple" were willing to receive help to pay their overdue electric bills.

In her last national revival tour, between September 1933 and December 20, 1934, two million persons heard 336 sermons. Many more were reached through 45 radio stations. A full crew of musicians, scene designers, and costumers accompanied McPherson.

In 1920, women were finally allowed to vote in the USA. It could be that McPherson had something to do with this, since she was known for empowering women. She was one of the most influential women in American history. Despite the scandals, negative news and outright hatred and criticism even from believers, she brought many to faith in Jesus Christ. Before the war, there were all-night prayer meetings held on Friday evenings. The pacifism, which had characterized the Foursquare denomination, was done away with. McPherson believed that one should fight for the freedoms America enjoyed. The amazing pouring out of the Holy Spirit in the Los Angeles area was the beginning of worldwide revival, which we know as the charismatic movement and is continuing to this day in various parts of the world.

"Foursquare" is an alternative word for "Full Gospel" (a term used by Pentecostals), referencing the nature of Christ's character: that he was Savior, Baptizer with the Holy Spirit, Healer, and soon-coming King. The four main beliefs were: the first being Christ's ability to transform individuals' lives through the act of salvation; the second focused on a holy baptism, which includes receiving power to glorify and exalt Christ in a practical way; the third was divine healing, newness of life for both body and spirit; and the fourth was gospel-oriented heed to the premillennial return of Jesus Christ.

1898-1984 John Peter Kolenda was an Assemblies of God missionary to Brazil and Germany. He also pastored churches in the USA, founded churches abroad, established Bible schools, started printing plants and taught extension courses.

Kolenda lived in Brazil from ages 4 to 11 before his family immigrated to the USA. At age 18, he was converted and began to read Maria Woodworth-Etter's *Signs and Wonders*. After this, through the ministry of Aimee Semple McPherson, he and other members of his family were filled with the Spirit and accepted divine healing.

He later went on to graduate from university, married and served as an evangelist for about six months, in Southern California. Later, he pastored churches in Michigan. He and his family arrived in

Brazil as missionaries when he was over 40 years old. He started over 100 churches or preaching points during the 14 years he ministered there. He took a furlough and when he returned, he taught at Bible conferences and served as superintendent of the work in the state of Santa Catarina. He began a monthly publication and provided Sunday school literature for the churches. During WW II, the mission work expanded considerably in South America. Later, Kolenda became a missionary in Germany for 10 years. He clearly shaped the Pentecostal movement in both Brazil and Germany.

John Peter Kolenda wasn't the only family member to make a large impact on the Pentecostal movement. One of John's older brothers, Paul, could easily have died a short time after his birth. He had a miracle recovery and went on to father ten sons. He was an Assemblies of God pastor in Illinois and Michigan. Most of these sons became preachers. One son, Daniel, is the president and CEO of Christ For All Nations, which was established by Evangelist Reinhard Bonnke.

1906-1973 Gordon Lindsay was a revivalist preacher, author, and founder of Christ for the Nations Institute.

Lindsay was born into a Pentecostal home. They were among the followers of John Dowie, a famous healing evangelist. Lindsay traveled with John Lake, who was campaigning in California and the southern states. He became an evangelist at age 18. He was associated with William Branham and they began a widely circulated magazine in 1948, called the "Voice of Healing." The magazine covered the ministries of other evangelists as well, such as Jack Coe, Oral Roberts and A.A. Allen. Lindsay wrote a biography of Branham in 1950. He also wrote 250 historical or doctrinal books on the healing revival movement.

Lindsay began sponsoring mission programs in several foreign countries and started a radio ministry. He sent teams of ministers around the world under the "Winning the Nations" crusade. His magazine name was changed to "Christ for the Nations." He wished to begin a Bible training institute. This materialized two years after his death. The Christ for the Nations Institute began in 1970, in Dallas, Texas and has trained thousands of students from around the world. As of 2018, there are 1200 students with 250 international students from 50 different nations. Lindsay's son is the current president.

The ministry has expanded to include a national church program, a national literature work, a Jewish mission in Israel, International Bible training schools and a prayer ministry.

He was the first evangelical writer to assume a link between the UFO phenomenon of our days and the fallen angels (Nephilim) in Genesis 6 and he has written books about this.

His daughter Shira is married to Pastor Ari Sorko-Ram, who founded the Maoz Israel ministry in Israel.

1907-1976 Kathryn Kuhlman was an American Pentecostal evangelist who was known for people receiving physical healings in her meetings.

Kuhlman had a spiritual experience at age 13 that changed her life. She was later ordained by the Evangelical Church Alliance and began to preach. She married a divorcee, but it was hardly a marriage and apparently lasted only about six years.

In the 1940's and 1970's, she traveled around the U.S. and other countries, holding "healing crusades." In the 1960s and 1970s, she had a weekly TV program as well as a 30-minute nationwide radio ministry of teaching. Key leaders of the Jesus movement, like David Wilkerson and Chuck Smith, endorsed her ministry.

By 1970, she moved to Los Angeles, conducting healing services for thousands of people each day as an heir to Aimee Semple McPherson. She became well known for her "gift of healing" despite, as she often noted, having no theological training. She was friends with Christian television pioneer Pat Robertson and made guest appearances at his *Christian Broadcasting Network (CBN)* and on the network's flagship program *The 700 Club*.

Her personal administrator once sued her for misuse of money, but Kuhlman stated that that everything was settled before going to trial.

Books were published about her ministry, one by a doctor, which was negative, and another which was positive. Jamie Buckingham wrote her biography. About two million people claimed to be healed in her meetings over the years.

In her late 40's she developed a heart problem, but still held meetings lasting from two to six hours. She later had open heart surgery, from which she died. She left a lot of money which went to three family members and twenty employees. Since she did not leave most of her estate to the foundation she founded (as she'd done in a previous will), they eventually had to discontinue the broadcasts in 1982. In 2016, the foundation closed its doors.

Her entire ministry was in question by many. She influenced faith healers Benny Hinn and Billy Burke. Martie Haaijer, a Dutch woman, traveled to the U.S. and was totally healed of cancer. After this, she began her own healing ministry in Holland and it was the first time people would "fall back" (attendants would always stand behind the people being prayed for). She passed away in 2008, at age 79.

1911-1970 Asa Alonso Allen better known as **A. A. Allen**, was an American Pentecostal evangelist known for his faith healing and deliverance ministry. He was, for a time, associated with the "Voice of Healing" movement founded by Gordon Lindsay.

Allen's parents were mixed; white and Native Americans. They were very poor and his father was an alcoholic. He was saved at the age of 23 in Missouri. Later he was baptized by the Holy Spirit when a Pentecostal preacher conducted meetings in their home. He felt called to preach and was ordained with the Assemblies of God church. He pastored in Colorado and in Texas. He attended Oral Robert's tent revival in 1949 and from this time he began his own divine healing ministry. He had a large following. He was one of the first to be on national television. He purchased a large tent. One tent which he used could seat over 22,000 people. He taught the prosperity gospel, expounding God's ability to perform financial miracles. At one time he appeared on fifty-eight radio stations daily, as well as forty-three television stations. A.A. Allen Revivals, Inc. was publishing over 60 million pieces of literature a year. His monthly "Miracle Magazine" was 450,000 at the time of his death. The magazine sometimes included accounts of healing, but the magazine didn't "assume legal responsibility" for their accuracy. Miracle Valley's annual payroll was $84,000. Allen did not like press coverage. Someone donated land to his ministry and they built Miracle Valley Bible College, a church, administrative buildings, a residential neighborhood, a printing plant and phonograph record plant. He divorced his wife. They had four children. Allen died at the age of 59 of liver failure. He unfortunately drank too much. He drank since he was in pain from arthritic bone spurs. He didn't seek a doctor since he believed in divine healing. He felt that relying on doctors was a failure to trust in G-d. Don Steward took over the property, moved it to Phoenix, Arizona and named it the Don Stewart Association. The Miracle Valley property was given to the Hispanic Assemblies and the Southern Arizona Bible College was founded. Part of this campus was destroyed by arson. It was rebuilt and was sold twenty years later. In 1982 there was a nasty law enforcement incident in which two church members were killed and multiple sheriff's deputies injured. Miracle Valley Bible College was purchased by Harter Ministries in 1999. The students studied Pentecostal theology, however the property was taken away. It was repurchased in 2011 by a non-denominational ministry called Miracle Valley Arizona Ministries. In 2014 another group purchased the property and plan to re-establish a Bible college.

…..- **1988 Lorne Fox** was healed and converted through the ministry of Charles Price. He was ordained with the Assemblies of G-d in 1934 and was a well-experienced pastor/evangelist when the Healing Revival broke out in 1947. He was quick to see what God was doing and began his own healing ministry with startling results. Associated with the 'Voice of Healing' he travelled worldwide to Europe, Africa and the Far East. Thousands came to Christ and experienced healing from Christ. One can obtain his book called *Visions of Heaven, Hell and the Cross.*

1918-2013 Harry Ararat Mushegan (Bishop) was a first-generation American whose parents narrowly escaped the Armenian genocide through their heeding of a prophetic warning (the same group of believers which included Demos Shakarian). He ministered in the Atlanta area for over five decades.

His descendants began the Ararat Church in 2019 which is in Smyrna, Georgia. It's interdenominational, multi-ethnic and full Gospel. There are three pastors; two male senior pastors and their mother, a founding pastor, together with another pastor. Salvation, healing and deliverance is taught.

1918-2009 Oral Roberts was an American Charismatic Christian televangelist, ordained in both the Pentecostal Holiness and United Methodist churches. He founded the Oral Roberts Evangelistic Association and Oral Roberts University.

Roberts was a descendant of Cherokee Indians. He began life in poverty and nearly died of tuberculosis at age 17. After college (he didn't receive the degree), he began to be a traveling faith healer. He had a tent which held 3,000 people. After preaching in churches for a short time, he began to hold crusades across the U.S. and around the world. He was guest speaker for many national and international meetings and conventions.

As one of the best-known and controversial American religious leaders of the 20th century, Roberts' preaching emphasized "seed-faith". His ministries reached millions of followers worldwide spanning a period of over six decades. His healing ministry and bringing American Pentecostalism into the mainstream had the most impact, but he also pioneered televangelism and laid the foundations of the prosperity gospel and abundant life teachings. The breadth and style of his ministry, including his widely publicized funding appeals, made him a consistent subject of contention among critics and supporters.

At its peak in the early 1980s, Roberts was the leader of a $120 million-a-year organization, employing 2,300 people. This spanned not only a university, but also a medical school and hospital (which was intended to merge medicine and prayer in the healing process), as well as buildings on 50 acres (200,000 m2) south of Tulsa, valued at $500 million. In 1965, students were admitted to the university. They were required to sign an honor code pledging not to drink, smoke, or engage in premarital sexual activities.

Roberts was a pioneer televangelist, and attracted a vast viewership. He was said to be second only to Billy Graham in popularity.

Roberts did have some money-raising drives which seemed to go wrong. He and his son are also said to have gotten involved in some scandals. Two out of four of Roberts' children died tragically.

+++

Worthy of mention are Ezekiel Guti in Zimbabwe and Mensah Otabil in Ghana. I have not included men which had a tarnished reputation, including William Branham.

A present-day ministry which you might be interested in is that of Dan Mohler. He can be found via google and youtube. In one message he told about a terrible headache he had for about a week. His wife kept trying to get him to go to a doctor. He refused. As he puts it, "In G-d's time it went away." Perhaps it was like a thorn in the flesh like Paul had.

GLEANINGS FROM THE GOSPELS

I made note of the following scriptures as I was reading through the New Testament while in the Italian Hospital. I've copied all of Luke 1 since I found it to be especially rich.

Matthew 28:17 - When they saw Him, they worshiped Him; but some doubted.

His 11 disciples KNEW Jesus and worshipped Him. How could any one of them doubt Jesus, seeing He had risen from the dead? The scripture makes it clear that some doubted. Even if some doubted the gospel message would continue to be propagated for the next 2,000 years.

Luke 1

Dedication to Theophilus

1 In as much as many have taken in hand to set in order
a narrative of those things which [a]have been fulfilled
among us, 2 just as those who from the beginning were
eyewitnesses and ministers of the word delivered them
to us, 3 it seemed good to me also, having [b]had perfect
understanding of all things from the very first, to write
to you an orderly account, most excellent Theophilus,
4 that you may know the certainty of those things in
which you were instructed.

John's Birth Announced to Zacharias

5 There was in the days of Herod, the king of Judea, a cer-
tain priest named Zacharias, of the division of Abijah. His
wife *was* of the daughters of Aaron, and her name *was*
Elizabeth. 6 And they were both righteous before God,
walking in all the commandments and ordinances of the
Lord blameless. 7 But they had no child, because Elizabeth
was barren, and they were both well advanced in years.

8 So it was, that while he was serving as priest before
God in the order of his division, 9 according to the cus-
tom of the priesthood, [c]his lot fell to burn incense when
he went into the temple of the Lord. 10 And the whole
multitude of the people was praying outside at the hour
of incense. 11 Then an angel of the Lord appeared to
him, standing on the right side of the altar of incense. 12
And when Zacharias saw *him,* he was troubled, and fear
fell upon him.

13 But the angel said to him, "Do not be afraid, Zach-
arias, for your prayer is heard; and your wife Elizabeth
will bear you a son, and you shall call his name John.
14 And you will have joy and gladness, and many will
rejoice at his birth. 15 For he will be great in the sight
of the Lord, and shall drink neither wine nor strong
drink. He will also be filled with the Holy Spirit, even
from his mother's womb. 16 And he will turn many of
the children of Israel to the Lord their God. 17 He will
also go before Him in the spirit and power of Elijah, 'to
turn the hearts of the fathers to the children,' and the
disobedient to the wisdom of the just, to make ready a
people prepared for the Lord."

18 And Zacharias said to the angel, "How shall I
know this? For I am an old man, and my wife is well
advanced in years."

19 And the angel answered and said to him, "I am
Gabriel, who stands in the presence of God, and was
sent to speak to you and bring you [d]these glad tidings.
20 But behold, you will be mute and not able to speak
until the day these things take place, because you did
not believe my words which will be fulfilled in their
own time."

21 And the people waited for Zacharias, and mar-
veled that he lingered so long in the temple. 22 But when
he came out, he could not speak to them; and they per-
ceived that he had seen a vision in the temple, for he
beckoned to them and remained speechless.

23 So it was, as soon as the days of his service were
completed, that he departed to his own house. 24 Now
after those days his wife Elizabeth conceived; and she
hid herself five months, saying, 25 "Thus the Lord has
dealt with me, in the days when He looked on *me,* to
take away my reproach among people."

Christ's Birth Announced to Mary

26 Now in the sixth month the angel Gabriel was sent
by God to a city of Galilee named Nazareth, 27 to a vir-
gin betrothed to a man whose name was Joseph, of the
house of David. The virgin's name *was* Mary. 28 And
having come in, the angel said to her, "Rejoice, highly
favored *one,* the Lord *is* with you; [e]blessed *are* you
among women!"

29 But [f]when she saw *him,* she was troubled at his
saying, and considered what manner of greeting this was.
30 Then the angel said to her, "Do not be afraid, Mary,
for you have found favor with God. 31 And behold, you
will conceive in your womb and bring forth a Son, and
shall call His name Jesus. 32 He will be great, and will be
called the Son of the Highest; and the Lord God will
give Him the throne of His father David. 33 And He
will reign over the house of Jacob forever, and of His
kingdom there will be no end."

34 Then Mary said to the angel, "How can this be,
since I [g]do not know a man?"

[35] And the angel answered and said to her, "*The*
Holy Spirit will come upon you, and the power of
the Highest will overshadow you; therefore, also, that
Holy One who is to be born will be called the Son of
God. [36] Now indeed, Elizabeth your relative has also
conceived a son in her old age; and this is now the
sixth month for her who was called barren. [37] For with
God nothing will be impossible."
[38] Then Mary said, "Behold the maidservant of the
Lord! Let it be to me according to your word." And the
angel departed from her.

Mary Visits Elizabeth

[39] Now Mary arose in those days and went into the hill
country with haste, to a city of Judah, [40] and entered
the house of Zacharias and greeted Elizabeth. [41] And it
happened, when Elizabeth heard the greeting of Mary,
that the babe leaped in her womb; and Elizabeth was
filled with the Holy Spirit. [42] Then she spoke out with
a loud voice and said, "Blessed *are* you among women,
and blessed *is* the fruit of your womb! [43] But why *is* this
granted to me, that the mother of my Lord should come
to me? [44] For indeed, as soon as the voice of your greet-
ing sounded in my ears, the babe leaped in my womb
for joy. [45] Blessed *is* she who [h]believed, for there will be
a fulfillment of those things which were told her from
the Lord."

The Song of Mary

46 And Mary said:

“My soul [i]magnifies the Lord,
47 And my spirit has rejoiced in God my Savior.
48 For He has regarded the lowly state of His maidservant;
For behold, henceforth all generations will call me blessed.
49 For He who is mighty has done great things for me,
And holy *is* His name.
50 And His mercy *is* on those who fear Him
From generation to generation.
51 He has shown strength with His arm;
He has scattered *the* proud in the imagination of their hearts.
52 He has put down the mighty from *their* thrones,
And exalted *the* lowly.
53 He has filled *the* hungry with good things,
And *the* rich He has sent away empty.
54 He has helped His servant Israel,
In remembrance of *His* mercy,
55 As He spoke to our fathers,
To Abraham and to his seed forever.”

56 And Mary remained with her about three months, and returned to her house.

Birth of John the Baptist

57 Now Elizabeth's full time came for her to be delivered, and she brought forth a son. 58 When her neighbors and relatives heard how the Lord had shown great mercy to her, they rejoiced with her.

Circumcision of John the Baptist

59 So it was, on the eighth day, that they came to circumcise the child; and they would have called him by the name of his father, Zacharias. 60 His mother answered and said, "No; he shall be called John."

61 But they said to her, "There is no one among your relatives who is called by this name." 62 So they made signs to his father—what he would have him called.

63 And he asked for a writing tablet, and wrote, saying, "His name is John." So they all marveled. 64 Immediately his mouth was opened and his tongue *loosed,* and he spoke, praising God. 65 Then fear came on all who dwelt around them; and all these sayings were discussed throughout all the hill country of Judea. 66 And all those who heard *them* kept *them* in their hearts, saying, "What kind of child will this be?" And the hand of the Lord was with him.

Zacharias' Prophecy

67 Now his father Zacharias was filled with the Holy Spirit, and prophesied, saying:

68 "Blessed *is* the Lord God of Israel,
For He has visited and redeemed His people,
69 And has raised up a horn of salvation for us
In the house of His servant David,
70 As He spoke by the mouth of His holy prophets,
Who *have been* since the world began,
71 That we should be saved from our enemies
And from the hand of all who hate us,
72 To perform the mercy *promised* to our fathers
And to remember His holy covenant,
73 The oath which He swore to our father Abraham:
74 To grant us that we,
Being delivered from the hand of our enemies,
Might serve Him without fear,
75 In holiness and righteousness before Him all the days of our life.
76 "And you, child, will be called the prophet of the Highest;
For you will go before the face of the Lord to prepare His ways,
77 To give knowledge of salvation to His people
By the remission of their sins,
78 Through the tender mercy of our God,
With which the [j]Dayspring from on high [k] has visited us;
79 To give light to those who sit in darkness and the shadow of death,
To guide our feet into the way of peace."

80 So the child grew and became strong in spirit, and was in the deserts till the day of his manifestation to Israel.

Footnotes

a. Luke 1:1 Or *are most surely believed*
b. Luke 1:3 Lit. *accurately followed*
c. Luke 1:9 *he was chosen by lot*
d. Luke 1:19 *this good news*
e. Luke 1:28 NU omits *blessed are you among women*
f. Luke 1:29 NU omits *when she saw him*
g. Luke 1:34 Am a virgin
h. Luke 1:45 Or *believed that there*
i. Luke 1:46 Declares the greatness of
j. Luke 1:78 Lit. *Dawn*; the Messiah
k. Luke 1:78 NU *shall visit*

Luke 1 is AMAZING!!!!!!!! Was my comment at the time. It is long and packed with very precious truths.

Luke 6:11 - But they were filled with rage, and discussed with one another what they might do to Jesus.

The scribes and Pharisees had set a trap for Jesus. He restored a man's withered hand. They were more concerned with their Sabbath observance than to see this man receive a miracle for which he had waited for many years. He would now be able to work.

Luke 8:53 - And they ridiculed Him, knowing that she was dead.

Jesus told those gathered around that they needed only to believe and the little girl would be made well. He also said not to weep; she is only sleeping. Jesus, his three disciples and the father and mother of the girl were permitted inside the house. Then Jesus went to where the girl was and called, "Little girl, arise." She came back to life and He commanded that she be given something to eat.

Luke 8:56 - And her parents were astonished, but He charged them to tell no one what had happened.

Don't you wonder why Jesus told the parents not to tell anyone? All in their immediate vicinity would see her about and surely ask. They would have no choice but to tell them that Jesus had raised her from the dead.

Luke 10:8 - Whatever city you enter, and they receive you, eat such things as are set before you.

What about missionaries in remote places who were offered strange food to eat? The Jewish people don't eat pork nor shell fish. What would they do? I read *Trusting Him,* by Robert A. Boomsma – the first book I read after the surgery about which I'm writing. He was in Myanmar and ate crickets from the open market. He was in many strange places but experienced stomach trouble only once. I must mention, however, that lately he has had to endure difficult surgeries. I wonder if it hadn't been better to stay away from something this exotic. It was not as if someone were offering it to him.

Luke 12:32 - Do not fear, little flock, for it is your Father's good pleasure to give you the kingdom.

What better assurance for these continuing Covid-19 days. We'll be here as long as our Heavenly father wants us to be here to promote His kingdom. We're not "kings" but rather a kingdom of priests. The original version of this verse in Revelation 1:6 must be translated properly.

Luke 19:5-6 - [5] And when Jesus came to the place, He looked up [NU omits and saw him] and saw him, and said to him, "Zacchaeus, [hurry] make haste and come down, for today I must stay at your house." [6] So he [hurried] made haste and came down, and received Him joyfully.

Isn't it wonderful to read about this successful Jewish businessman who had a heart for Jesus?

Luke 21:15 - for I will give you a mouth and wisdom which all your adversaries will not be able to contradict or [withstand] resist.

Dear Lord, this is what I want and need. I accept this promise which is still relevant and valid.

Luke 21:35 - For it will come as a snare on all those who dwell on the face of the whole earth.

What is the snare? The snare is listed in the previous verse. It's what's weighing our hearts down; carousing, drunkenness and care of this life. We must PRAY ALWAYS (the verse following) to be counted worthy to escape these things that will come to pass and to stand before the Son of man.

Luke 22:15 - Then He said to them, "With *fervent* desire I have desired to eat this Passover with you before I suffer;

Jesus loved His disciples very much. Don't you find it amazing that apart from one, the eleven stuck with their rabbi for three years. They didn't leave to return to their families. Would they have sent a letter home from time to time? People DID write letters in those times (Paul wrote even some long ones!). Would they have sent a messenger with some cash to their wives and families? When they were in Tiberias and had the great fishing success, would part of the catch have gone to their nearby families? The Bible is inspired. It's G-d's own words through the writers and is our guide book. It's not filled with unnecessary details. Who agrees?

Luke 22:22 - And truly the Son of Man goes as it has been determined, but woe to that man by whom He is betrayed!

Judas had a tremendous burden on himself. This is what caused him to commit suicide; he had betrayed the sinless Son of Man and Son of G-d.

Luke 22:28-29 - But you are those who have continued with Me in My trials. 29 And I bestow upon you a kingdom, just as My Father bestowed *one* upon Me,

Kingdom business doesn't come without trials, my dear readers. Trials strengthen our faith. Trials build our character. 2 Corinthians 1:4-7 assures us that when we're going through tough circumstances, this will enable us to identify and share in other people's sufferings. Perhaps Paul's "thorn in the flesh" kept him humble and more understanding of those he came across who suffered from one thing or another.

Luke 22:32 - But I have prayed for you, that your faith should not fail; and when you have returned to *Me,* strengthen your brethren.

Peter had failed the Lord but thankfully he returned to the Lord and to his calling. Not only did Jesus pray for him; He prays for all of us from His throne. Hebrews 7:25b says, "He always lives to make intercession for them." This is speaking of our Jesus as a priest who is sitting at G-d's right hand.

Luke 22:37 - For I say to you that this which is written must still be [fulfilled] accomplished in Me: 'And He was numbered with the transgressors.' For the things concerning Me have an end.

Jesus cried "It is finished" when He was hanging on the cross. He told his disciples this while giving some instructions for their future evangelistic work. These few men would change the world within a rather small space of time. Remember that when they preached, they taught and talked of both His death and His resurrection. Both must be presented. Jesus atoned for our sins through the shedding of His precious blood. He rose after three days and nights. He had victory over death; so will we. Of course, we'll die like everyone else but not eternally. Our soul and spirit live on forever and we'll have a new glorified body like Jesus had after His resurrection. The resurrection power needs to be taught. Paul states in Philippians 3:10 that I may know Him and the power of His resurrection, and the fellowship of His sufferings, being conformed to His death.

Luke 22:43 - Then an angel appeared to Him from heaven, strengthening Him. (this verse not in original text?)

This was when he was praying in the garden that the cup would pass from him.

Luke 22:51 - But Jesus answered and said, "Permit even this." And He touched his ear and healed him.

One of the disciples cut the high priest's servant's ear off with a sword. Jesus immediately touched it and it was restored. John tells us that this disciple was Simon Peter.

Luke 22:53 - When I was with you daily in the temple, you did not try to seize Me. But this is your hour, and the power of darkness.

Do you wonder why Jesus said this?

Luke 23:27 - And a great multitude of the people followed Him, and women who also mourned and lamented Him.

The famous movies showing Jesus being taken to be crucified get this right. They always show a crowd. The disciples had fled but the crowd was watching, except for at least John who was there at the cross.

John 2:15 - When He had made a whip of cords, He drove them all out of the temple, with the sheep and the oxen, and poured out the changers' money and overturned the tables.

Small cords? It says this in one of the translations. Small cords against a few pigeons or people could also do the job. Righteous indignation. I think the believers need some of this because of this passage in Hebrews 12:4. You have not yet resisted to bloodshed, striving against sin.

Charles Clarke wrote *Pioneers of Revival* in 1971. He writes about William Booth who founded the Salvation Army. Here is a description of one of their bold activities. "Terrible evils lay hidden under the curtain of Victorian social life in the nineteenth century. The Salvation Army unmasked and fought them. Its work among prostitutes soon revealed the appalling wickedness of the white slave traffic, in which girls of thirteen were sold by their parents to the pimps who used them in their profitable brothels, or who traded them on the Continent.

Thousands of innocent girls, most of them under sixteen, were shipped as regularly as cattle to the state-regulated brothels of Brussels and Antwerp' (Collier)."

In another section of the chapter he writes as follows: "As the work of the Salvation Army spread throughout Britain and into many countries overseas, it met with brutal hostility. In many places Skeleton Armies were organized to sabotage this work of God. Hundreds of officers were attacked and injured (some for life). Halls and offices were smashed and fired. Meetings were broken up by gangs organized by brothel keepers and hostile publicans. One sympathizer in Worthing defended his life and property with a revolver. But Booth's soldiers endured the persecution for many years, often winning over their opponents by their own offensive of Christian love."

John 5:5 - Now a certain man was there who had an infirmity thirty-eight years.

Half a life-time...

John 5:14 - Afterward Jesus found him in the temple, and said to him, "See, you have been made well. Sin no more, lest a worse thing come upon you."

Jesus looked for him in order to encourage him; also to warn him to stay on the path of believing in Him.

John 6:15 - Therefore when Jesus perceived that they were about to come and take Him by force to make Him king, He departed again to the mountain by Himself alone.

We need the Holy Spirit's promptings. We need to know when to move on. John 10:27 My sheep hear My voice, and I know them, and they follow Me.

John 6:51 - I am the living bread which came down from heaven. If anyone eats of this bread, he will live forever; and the bread that I shall give is My flesh, which I shall give for the life of the world.

The whole world needs this bread. Bread is very different in various parts of the world. In rice-consuming countries, even if they don't eat bread, they would know that it is the most essential food for life.

John 6:54 - Whoever eats My flesh and drinks My blood has eternal life, and I will raise him up at the last day.

We need to partake of the bread and wine frequently in remembrance of what Jesus has done for us. 1 Corinthians 11:25-26 In the same manner *He* also *took* the cup after supper, saying, "This cup is the new covenant in My blood. This do, as often as you drink *it*, in remembrance of Me." 26 For as often as you eat this bread and drink this cup, you proclaim the Lord's death till He comes.

John 6:66 - From that *time* many of His disciples went [away or to the back] back and walked with Him no more

This is one of the saddest verses in the Bible. Jesus had invested a lot in their lives. They were leaving because of what is written in John 6:63 "It is the Spirit who gives life; the flesh profits nothing. The words that I speak to you are spirit, and *they* are life." They want to mix something of their own initiative when it came to carrying out their commission. Have you heard about Mr. Willing and Mr. Able? There are those who might be more able to an assignment but who aren't willing. Perhaps G-d uses the less capable or gifted to do a job. They will be more inclined to do the job right since it will be the Holy Spirit working in and through them.

John 7:20 - The people answered and said, "You have a demon. Who is seeking to kill You?"

Jesus shows up in the middle of the Feast of Tabernacles in Jerusalem. The people were seeking Him out since there was a LOT of complaining about Him among the Jews. He said that if anyone wants to do G-d's will, he would know whether or not I'm speaking from G-d's authority or my own. One who speaks from himself seeks his own glory; but He who seeks the glory of the One who sent Him is true, and no unrighteousness is in Him. As if this isn't enough, He pricks them when He says, "Did not Moses give you the law, yet NONE of you keeps the law? Why do you seek to kill Me?"

John 7:26 - But look! He speaks boldly, and they say nothing to Him. Do the rulers know indeed that this is [NU omits truly] truly the Christ?

Jesus continues on with bold words. They circumcise on the Sabbath so why shouldn't He have made a man whole on the Sabbath? He claims that G-d who sent Him is true. Again He says they do not know Him.

John 7:31 - And many of the people believed in Him, and said, "When the Christ comes, will He do more signs than these which this *Man* has done?"

How wonderful that MANY of them believed on Him. The one who seeks will always find. This promise is found in Jeremiah 29:13 And you will seek Me and find *Me,* when you search for Me with all your heart.

John 7:33 - Then Jesus said [NU, M omit "to them"] to them, "I shall be with you a little while longer, and *then* I go to Him who sent Me.

Jesus's ministry lasted a short three years.

John 8:21 - Then Jesus said to them again, "I am going away, and you will seek Me, and will die in your sin. Where I go you cannot come."

Jesus will soon go to the father G-d. Those of us who have received Him as savior will see Him after we die. Not only do we have hope in this life with the guidance of the Holy Spirit in every aspect (as long as we're obedience children!); we have hope of eternal life in a brand new world in which there is no sorrow, nor pain. It will be a huge international gathering without parallel on this side of heaven. We will all be able to speak to one another in a common language. I'm really looking forward to this. I'm also looking forward to meeting the Bible heroes and asking them questions. Who will you look for, after seeing Jesus face to face?

John 8:25 - Then they said to Him, "Who are You?"

And Jesus said to them, "Just what I have been saying to you from the beginning.

He has much to say and He can judge those He's talking to but He will speak only what He's heard from the Father. Again many people believed in Him.

I could elaborate more here but I am being true to the verses which I noted while in the hospital!

John 9:16 - Therefore some of the Pharisees said, "This Man is not from God, because He does not [observe] keep the Sabbath."

Others said, "How can a man who is a sinner do such signs?" And there was a division among them.

Jesus healed the blind man who was blind from birth. They couldn't understand that Jesus was greater than their Jewish laws and traditions.

John 9:18 - But the Jews did not believe concerning him, that he had been blind and received his sight, until they called the parents of him who had received his sight.

In this case, to our surprise, "Seeing was not believing." They saw a man whom they knew was blind for many years, yet they had to confirm the miracle by talking with his parents.

John 9:22 - His parents said these *things* because they feared the Jews, for the Jews had agreed already that if anyone confessed *that* He *was* Christ, he would be put out of the synagogue.

His parents avoided answering the question as to who opened his eyes and told them to ask the man himself since he was old enough to explain what happened. Do we see here how important the synagogue was to these people? How necessary would it be if Jesus was offering them a completely new and better way of life?

John 9:25 - He answered and said, "Whether He is a sinner *or not* I do not know. One thing I know: that though I was blind, now I see."

The former blind man gave an honest answer.

John 9:27 - He answered them, "I told you already, and you did not listen. Why do you want to hear *it* again? Do you also want to become His disciples?"

Ouch! The questioners weren't being nice to him, nor were they open to realize the supernatural which had occurred here.

John 9:31 - Now we know that God does not hear sinners; but if anyone is a worshiper of God and does His will, He hears him.

Who says G-d doesn't hear sinners? He's a "babe" in Christ. Here we have the distinction made between a life of religion and works as opposed to receiving the free gift of salvation. From this point the blind man has been born again but he needs to understand what has happened. When Jesus tells Nicodemus in John 3 how he must be born from above, he understands.

John 9:33-35 - If this Man were not from God, He could do nothing."[34] They answered and said to him, "You were completely born in sins, and are you teaching us?" And they [excommunicated him] cast him out.[35] Jesus heard that they had cast him out; and when He had found him, He said to him, "Do you believe in the Son of [NU Man] God?"

These religious folks were stamping out a small light of hope but in fact a blind man receiving his sight is something irretractable and amazing. He will never be the same. Jesus, being all-knowing, came and rescued him from any doubt.

John 9:39 - And Jesus said, "For judgment I have come into this world, that those who do not see may see, and that those who see may be made blind."

If we remember this, we shouldn't be surprised that so many self-righteous, successful, rich or important people don't believe in Jesus. We're aware that many of those types are not called from 1 Corinthians 1:26 For [consider] you see your calling, brethren, that not many wise according to the flesh, not many mighty, not many [well-born] noble, *are called.*

John 10:21 - Others said, "These are not the words of one who has a demon. Can a demon open the eyes of the blind?"

Jesus had just finished teaching them about the sheep following the shepherd. Many sheep could be lost or destroyed by the wolf if they're not in the shepherd's care. He's only telling the truth about Himself but there was a division among the Jews. They bring up the subject of the healing of the blind man. They're not used to the supernatural. Those who truly belong to those His father has given to Him will not be taken out of His hand. He is claiming here to be one with His Father, and therefore G-d. Look at their reaction immediately below.

John 10: 31 - Then the Jews took up stones again to stone Him.

Jesus asks them for what they're stoning Him. They accuse Him of blasphemy.

John 10:38-39 - but if I do, though you do not believe Me, believe the works, that you may know and [understand] believe that the Father *is* in Me, and I in Him." [39] Therefore they sought again to seize Him, but He escaped out of their hand.

G-d saw to it that He escaped. It was not yet His time to be captured.

John 11:16 - Then Thomas, who is called the Twin, said to his fellow disciples, "Let us also go, that we may die with Him."

They're on their way to visit Lazarus. Thomas – enough negative talk! Why would he say that?

John 11:28 - And when she had said these things, she went her way and secretly called Mary her sister, saying, "The Teacher has come and is calling for you."

Martha actually made this up – take a look! Perhaps it triggered her subsequent behavior, however. Later she listened at his feet. Maybe we should use this tactic with an unsaved friend? It's not a lie in that Jesus is calling for all people to come to Him.

John 11:40 - Jesus said to her, "Did I not say to you that if you would believe you would see the glory of God?"

Martha was reminding the Lord that there was a terrible smell inside since Lazarus had already been dead for four days.

John 11:48 - If we let Him alone like this, everyone will believe in Him, and the Romans will come and take away both our place and nation."

MANY of the Jews had been to the location of Lazarus's rising from the dead but they didn't believe and were fearful that the news would spread far and wide. They were afraid of the change in their status quo.

John 11:52 - and not for that nation only, but also that He would gather together in one the children of God who were scattered abroad.

Caiaphas, the high priest prophesied that Jesus would die for the nation. The second part of this prophecy would be fulfilled more than 2,000 years later. This is the age in which we're now alive and the Jewish people who are scattered abroad are coming home in greater numbers than ever before. This is referring to those of the Jewish nation but also to those who are sons of Abraham by faith; the family of G-d made up of Jew and Gentile.

John 12:37 - But although He had done so many signs before them, they did not believe in Him,

Would we be any different today? In the last days there will be some miracles but which aren't truly from G-d. Matthew 7:22-23 Many will say to Me in that day, 'Lord, Lord, have we not prophesied in Your name, cast out demons in Your name, and done many wonders in Your name?' 23 And then I will declare to them, 'I never knew you; depart from Me, you who practice lawlessness!'

John 17:14 - I have given them Your word; and the world has hated them because they are not of the world, just as I am not of the world.

If Jesus and His people were hated, so shall we be hated who stand for all that He stands for.

John 18:8 - Jesus answered, "I have told you that I am *He.* Therefore, if you seek Me, let these go their way,"

Jesus is being arrested in the garden at the Mount of Olives. He is actually dismissing his disciples here who had been with Him. He will go with the officers who came to arrest Him without resistance.

John 18:20 - Jesus answered him, "I spoke openly to the world. I always taught in synagogues and in the temple, where [*NU all the Jews meet*] the Jews always meet, and in secret I have said nothing.

Jesus was speaking to the high priest. He said that he could ask those who have heard His teachings. One of the officers hit Jesus with the palm of his hand after he said this and said, "Do you answer the high priest like that?" After this He was bound and sent to Caiaphas.

John 20:27 - Then He said to Thomas, "Reach your finger here, and look at My hands; and reach your hand *here,* and put *it* into My side. Do not be unbelieving, but believing.

After this Thomas believed. He said, "My Lord and my G-d!" Jesus said, "Blessed are those who have not seen and yet have believed."

John 21:23 - Then this saying went out among the brethren that this disciple would not die. Yet Jesus did not say to him that he would not die, but, "If I will that he remain till I come, what *is that* to you?

Peter was wondering about John. After this some of the believers thought that John would not die. Jesus did not say this, however, but rather that if so, what is it to you?

Acts 2:5 - And there were dwelling in Jerusalem Jews, devout men, from every nation under heaven.

They managed to come without modern transportation.

GLEANINGS FROM ACTS AND ROMANS

Acts 2:39-40 - For the promise is to you and to your children, and to all who are afar off, as many as the Lord our God will call." 40 And with many other words he testified and exhorted them, saying, "Be saved from this [crooked] perverse generation."

I would guess that our generation is far more perverse.

Acts 2:43 - Then fear came upon every soul, and many wonders and signs were done through the apostles.

The Holy Spirit had been poured out on the disciples. They were doing the miracles like Jesus had done. This is supposed to be the pattern to this day. Why? Because Jesus said so in John 14:12 "Most assuredly, I say to you, he who believes in Me, the works that I do he will do also; and greater *works* than these he will do, because I go to My Father."

Acts 2:47 - praising God and having favor with all the people. And the Lord added [NU omits "to the church] to the church daily those who were being saved.

Peter's sermon in Jerusalem had great results; three thousand souls. Here was a healthy, growing, caring church which was expanding with new believers in Jesus. The opposition comes later. This was a wonderful time for people to get grounded in their newfound faith.

Acts 3:2 - And a certain man lame from his mother's womb was carried, whom they laid daily at the gate of the temple which is called Beautiful, to [beg] ask alms from those who entered the temple;

G-d used Peter and John to heal this man. He began leaping and praising G-d. What a spectacle as he entered the temple in this way!

Acts 3:7-8 - And he took him by the right hand and lifted *him* up, and immediately his feet and ankle bones received strength. [8] So he, leaping up, stood and walked and entered the temple with them—walking, leaping, and praising God.

Acts 3:11 - Now as the lame man who was healed held on to Peter and John, all the people ran together to them in the porch which is called Solomon's, greatly amazed.

All the people ran to see what was happening. Of course, Peter immediately denies taking credit for the miracle and gives them a pointed sermon about how THEY delivered Jesus up to Pilate. You requested that a murderer be saved instead of Jesus. You were ignorant as well as your rulers, but he stresses that Jesus arose from the dead.

Acts 3:26 - To you first, God, having raised up His Servant Jesus, sent Him to bless you, in turning away every one *of you* from your iniquities."

Jesus doesn't want to condemn, but to save. He wants to bless. Remember John 3:17? For God did not send His Son into the world to condemn the world, but that the world through Him might be saved.

Acts 4:21 - So when they had further threatened them, they let them go, finding no way of punishing them, because of the people, since they all glorified God for what had been done.

This time they were freed.

Acts 4:31 - And when they had prayed, the place where they were assembled together was shaken; and they were all filled with the Holy Spirit, and they spoke the word of God with boldness.

Peter and John prayed for those who were threatening them and asked for boldness to speak G-d's word. This was a prayer meeting in which ALL were filled with the Holy Spirit and they spoke the word of G-d with boldness.

Acts 5:20 - "Go, stand in the temple and speak to the people all the words of this life."

They were eventually imprisoned but the angel brought them out and told them to continue preaching, which they did.

Acts 5:29 - But Peter and the *other* apostles answered and said: "We ought to obey God rather than men.

The captain and officers caught them preaching again in the temple. Peter and the apostles were obeying a higher authority than the Roman rulers.

Acts 5:31 - Him God has exalted to His right hand *to be* Prince and Savior, to give repentance to Israel and forgiveness of sins.

Jesus has accomplished this for everyone.

Acts 7:9 - And the patriarchs, becoming envious, sold Joseph into Egypt. But God was with him

Both Jesus and Joseph had been humiliated (and this is an understatement) before they were exalted.

Acts 8:21 - You have neither part nor portion in this matter, for your heart is not right in the sight of God.

Simon was a sorcerer and thought he could buy the power of G-d. He did ask for prayer.

Acts 8:29 - Then the Spirit said to Philip, "Go near and overtake this chariot."

If we're sensitive to the voice of the Holy Spirit, He'll tell us where to go.

Acts 8:40 - But Philip was found at [Ashdod]Azotus. And passing through, he preached in all the cities till he came to Caesarea.

Have you heard of "Philip transportation?" He baptized his new convert and afterwards supernaturally arrived at the next location where he was needed.

Acts 9:15 - But the Lord said to him, "Go, for he is a chosen vessel of Mine to bear My name before Gentiles, kings, and the children[sons] of Israel."

Ananias knew that Saul had been seeking out Christians to kill them. After hearing the Lord, he obeyed.

Acts 9:24 - But their plot became known to Saul. And they watched the gates day and night, to kill him.

G-d is our deliverer. The scriptures are full of those He delivered, both in the Old Testament and the New. Don't we love the stories of Abraham, Isaac, Joseph, Moses, Daniel and the 3 Hebrews, Esther, David, Jeremiah and others? And the WHOLE nation of Israel was delivered miraculously from the fierce army of Pharaoh, which G-d COMPLETELY destroyed in the Red Sea.

Acts 9:26 - And when Saul had come to Jerusalem, he tried to join the disciples; but they were all afraid of him, and did not believe that he was a disciple.

Who could blame them? One must have discernment! Thankfully Barnabas knew the facts and calmed them down.

Acts 9:35 - So all who dwelt at Lydda and Sharon saw him and turned to the Lord.

A poor paralyzed man, bedridden for eight years was healed. Would that we would see these miracles today; many more would be saved.

Acts 9:40 - But Peter put them all out, and knelt down and prayed. And turning to the body he said, "Tabitha, arise." And she opened her eyes, and when she saw Peter she sat up.

Dorcas was a seamstress who had died. G-d used Peter to raise her up and MANY in Joppa believed on the Lord. He stayed there many days.

Acts 9:43 - So it was that he stayed many days in Joppa with Simon, a tanner.

This is called "follow-up." It's necessary to make sure that new believers understand the basics about their faith.

Acts 10:15 - And a voice *spoke* to him again the second time, "What God has [declared clean] cleansed you must not call common."

He was terribly conflicted since as a Jew he would never eat non-kosher food. I don't think this is a passage to justify eating non-kosher food but that's just my humble understanding. My husband and I are living in Israel since the late 70's and we don't eat pork or any type of shell fish. I personally it's healthier to be without them. If our children choose a different way, it's their decision.

Acts 10:23 - Then he invited them in and lodged *them.* On the next day Peter went away with them, and some brethren from Joppa accompanied him.

Cornelius was INSTRUCTED by a holy angel to invite Peter to come and teach him. Would we believe a non-believer if they told us this? Hospitality – something traditional for hundreds of years in the Middle East.

Acts 10:27 - And as he talked with him, he went in and found many who had come together.

Prayer preparation before evangelistic services or any type of outreach is needed to "prepare the hearts."

Acts 10:33 - So I sent to you immediately, and you have done well to come. Now therefore, we are all present before God, to hear all the things commanded you by God.

When Adoniran Judson went to Burma he discovered the Karen folks already anticipated a white man to bring a "lost book" to them. It was seven years before the first convert, who was a former killer. His conversion was a very important key in the salvation of many. There were many hindrances in the translation work but Judson will have a sure reward in heaven.

Acts 10:43 - To Him all the prophets witness that, through His name, whoever believes in Him will receive remission[forgiveness] of sins.

Had these Jewish people studied their scriptures they would have seen Jesus already on many pages of the prophets. Are we studying our scriptures?

Acts 10:48 - And he commanded them to be baptized in the name of the Lord. Then they asked him to stay a few days.

Baptismal service – how wonderful. Then "follow-up!"

Acts 11:28 - Then one of them, named Agabus, stood up and showed by the Spirit that there was going to be a great famine throughout all the world, which also happened in the days of Claudius Caesar.

Can we believe our modern day prophets? This man prophesied in order that the folks would prepare themselves, in the same way Joseph prophesied of famine in Egypt.

Acts 12:5 - Peter was therefore kept in prison, but [NU *constantly* or *earnestly*] constant prayer was offered to God for him by the church.

Such a preacher would stir up trouble in time. Paul made good use of his time in prison, writing many, many pages.

Acts 12:16 - Now Peter continued knocking; and when they opened *the door* and saw him, they were astonished.

Poor Rhoda – she gets the blame but shouldn't since Paul writes that because of her gladness she left him standing there. He went in and explained his marvelous escape from the prison but then moved on. Herod wanted him dead!

Acts 12:19 - But when Herod had searched for him and not found him, he examined the guards and commanded that *they* should be put to death.

And he went down from Judea to Caesarea, and stayed *there.*

G-d still had work for Paul to do so He protected him on his trip out of Judea. His prison guards were apparently killed. It probably says "down to Caesarea" since when it comes to Jerusalem we always go "up." Jerusalem is in Judea.

Acts 12:22-24 - And the people kept shouting, "The voice of a god and not of a man!" 23 Then immediately an angel of the Lord struck him, because he did not give glory to God. And he was eaten by worms and [breathed his last] died. 24 But the word of God grew and multiplied.

BUT – don't you love this! Would to G-d that some folks would be struck down due to their evil ways and pride.

Acts 13:8 - But Elymas the sorcerer (for so his name is translated) [opposed] withstood them, seeking to turn the proconsul away from the faith.

Acts 13:11 – "And now, indeed, the hand of the Lord *is* upon you, and you shall be blind, not seeing the sun for a time." And immediately a dark mist fell on him, and he went around seeking someone to lead him by the hand.

G-d's power was manifested. Paul called him out for his perversion of the ways of the Lord. He became blind for a time.

Acts 13:34 - And that He raised Him from the dead, no more to return to [the state of decay] corruption, He has spoken thus:

'I will give you the sure [blessings] mercies of David.'

Paul's powerful recorded sermon in Antioch in the synagogue.

> Acts 13:41 - 'Behold, you despisers,
> Marvel and perish!
> For I work a work in your days,
> A work which you will by no means believe,
> Though one were to declare it to you.' "

Many of the Jews were persuaded and wished to continue with Paul after this service. The Gentiles wanted to hear the same sermon preached to them the following week.

Acts 13:46 - Then Paul and Barnabas grew bold and said, "It was necessary that the word of God should be spoken to you first; but since you reject it, and judge yourselves unworthy of everlasting life, behold, we turn to the Gentiles."

Watershed moment. What I always found interesting was that the preacher for the Jews was the uneducated fisherman, Peter, and Paul, the great Jewish expert in all Jewish law and practice would go to the Gentiles.

Acts 13:48-52 - Now when the Gentiles heard this, they were glad and glorified the word of the Lord. And as many as had been appointed to eternal life believed. [49] And the word of the Lord was being spread throughout all the region. [50] But the Jews stirred up the devout and prominent women and the chief men of the city, raised up persecution against Paul and Barnabas, and expelled them from their region. [51] But they shook off the dust from their feet against them, and came to Iconium. [52] And the disciples were filled with joy and with the Holy Spirit.

Jesus had said to move along if the people in a given place don't receive you. There are always seeking souls somewhere in the world.

Acts 14:2 - But the unbelieving Jews stirred up the Gentiles and [embittered] poisoned their [souls] minds against the brethren.

They reacted in an unusual way, however; namely, THEREFORE, they stayed there a long time! (verse 3) Signs and wonders were seen.

Acts 14:5 - And when a violent attempt was made by both the Gentiles and Jews, with their rulers, to abuse and stone them,

G-d warned them and they left in time.

Acts 14:9-10 - *This* man heard Paul speaking. [Who] Paul, observing him intently and seeing that he had faith to be healed, 10 said with a loud voice, "Stand up straight on your feet!" And he leaped and walked.

G-d gives discernment to those with a gift of healing. I've heard many stories – also some true incidents which occurred via the TV ministries. Nowadays we're speaking of online. G-d's not limited, of course.

Acts 15:39 - Then the contention became so sharp that they parted from one another. And so Barnabas took Mark and sailed to Cyprus;

OK – it happens to the best of them… and to this day.

Acts 16:14 - Now a certain woman named Lydia heard *us.* She was a seller of purple from the city of Thyatira, who worshiped God. The Lord opened her heart to heed the things spoken by Paul.

An entrepreneur. We need more present day women doing enterprising things. Even Proverbs 31 talks about an enterprising woman.

Acts 16:18 - And this she did for many days. But Paul, greatly [distressed] annoyed, turned and said to the spirit, "I command you in the name of Jesus Christ to come out of her." And he came out that very hour.

Paul, after many days became GREATLY ANNOYED. I'm surprised he waited so long. Perhaps it was like good advertising. Sometimes when there are negative articles about a certain ministry, it gets people's attention – maybe non-believing readers even check something out. Praise G-d she was delivered.

Acts 16:24 - Having received such a charge, he put them into the inner prison and fastened their feet in the stocks.

Paul and Silas are silenced for now.

Acts 16:37 - But Paul said to them, "They have beaten us openly, uncondemned Romans, *and* have thrown *us* into prison. And now do they put us out secretly? No indeed! Let them come themselves and get us out."

This is interesting. Have you wondered about this? I would make interesting media coverage in our times.

Acts 17:6 - But when they did not find them, they dragged Jason and some brethren to the rulers of the city, crying out, "These who have turned the world upside down have come here too.

What a beautiful charge – would that someone would turn our world upside down with the good news of the gospel somewhere/anywhere in our world. Jason, who was housing them suffered a great deal due to his hospitality. I'm thankful for all of the righteous Gentiles who hid the Jewish people during WW II, like the Ten Boom family.

Acts 17:11 - These were more [noble] fair-minded than those in Thessalonica, in that they received the word with all readiness, and searched the Scriptures daily *to find out* whether these things were so.

We can never study the Bible too much. Even a pastor is a human being and may need some correction here and there but if so, it should be given "in love."

Acts 17:16 - Now while Paul waited for them at Athens, his spirit was provoked within him when he saw that the city was [full of idols] given over to idols.

Are we provoked when we see evil around us?

Acts 17:21 - For all the Athenians and the foreigners who were there spent their time in nothing else but either to tell or to hear some new thing.

Better to get a job or write a book instead of just "shooting the breeze" (my American expression for wasting time with unimportant conversations).

Acts 17:27 - so that they should seek the Lord, in the hope that they might grope for Him and find Him, though He is not far from each one of us;

Psalm 145:18 The Lord *is* near to all who call upon Him, To all who call upon Him in truth.

Acts 17:31 - because He has appointed a day on which He will judge the world in righteousness by the Man whom He has ordained. He has given assurance of this to all by raising Him from the dead.

I would be amazed if a person doesn't think there will eventually be a day of accounting for how one spent his/her life. I would guess it's in the major religions for starters.

Acts 18:2 - And he found a certain Jew named Aquila, born in Pontus, who had recently come from Italy with his wife Priscilla (because Claudius had commanded all the Jews to depart from Rome); and he came to them.

They made "aliyah" to Israel! They started a joint venture with tentmaker Paul.

Acts 18:6 - But when they opposed him and blasphemed, he shook *his* garments and said to them, "Your blood *be* upon your *own* heads; I *am* clean. From now on I will go to the Gentiles."

There are others to whom to preach – he moved on.

Acts 18:10 - for I am with you, and no one will attack you to hurt you; for I have many people in this city.

He was told by G-d to stay in that same city but no one would attack him anymore.

Acts 19:6 - And when Paul had laid hands on them, the Holy Spirit came upon them, and they spoke with tongues and prophesied.

Paul is now in Ephesus. This is a good formula to this day. I won't go into details here.

Acts 19:9-10 - But when some were hardened and did not believe, but spoke evil of the Way before the multitude, he departed from them and withdrew the disciples, reasoning daily in the school of Tyrannus. [10] And this continued for two years, so that all who dwelt in Asia heard the word of the Lord Jesus, both Jews and Greeks.

When there was opposition he moved on. ALL heard it says… (and this without electronic means!).

Acts 19:16 - Then the man in whom the evil spirit was leaped on them, [M and they overpowered them] overpowered them, and prevailed against [NU both of them] them, so that they fled out of that house naked and wounded.

This is a sobering passage. When dealing with evil spirits, much godly wisdom is required.

Acts 19:37 - For you have brought these men here who are neither robbers of temples nor blasphemers of [NU our] your goddess.

He demanded order of the people in Ephesus. If there is a case against Paul, it should be bought before the courts.

Acts 20:24 – [NU But I do not count my life of any value or dear to myself] But none of these things move me; nor do I count my life dear to myself, so that I may finish my [course] race with joy, and the ministry which I received from the Lord Jesus, to testify to the gospel of the grace of God.

Do we count our lives dear unto ourselves? The famous missionary to the Aucas, Jim Elliot said, "He is no fool who gives what he cannot keep to gain what he cannot lose."

Acts 20:28 - Therefore take heed to yourselves and to all the flock, among which the Holy Spirit has made you overseers, to shepherd the church [M of the Lord and God] of God which He purchased with His own blood.

Paul in Ephesus is warning the believers of the need to oversee the church well since wolves will come in afterwards. Their faith will be tested.

Acts 20:31 - Therefore watch, and remember that for three years I did not cease to warn everyone night and day with tears.

Tears? Do I know any Shepherd who is warning people with tears? Yes, actually Georgian Banov… He knows the evils of Communism since he saw it first hand in Bulgaria. He prays more fervently than anyone I know for his adopted country of America.

Acts 21:4 - And finding [NU the disciples] disciples, we stayed there seven days. They told Paul through the Spirit not to go up to Jerusalem.

Did he listen, however?

Acts 21:31-32 - Now as they were seeking to kill him, news came to the commander of the [cohort] garrison that all Jerusalem was in an uproar. 32 He immediately took soldiers and centurions, and ran down to them. And when they saw the commander and the soldiers, they stopped beating Paul.

He was caught but afterwards gave a VERY LONG sermon to many people.

Acts 22:14-15 - Then he said, 'The God of our fathers has chosen you that you should know His will, and see the Just One, and hear the voice of His mouth. 15 For you will be His witness to all men of what you have seen and heard.

G-d chose a dangerous rebel who was out to officially kill the believers in Jesus.

Acts 23:5 - Then Paul said, "I did not know, brethren, that he was the high priest; for it is written, 'You shall not speak evil of a ruler of your people.'"

He knew the scripture and also apologized, which was appropriate.

Acts 23:22 - So the commander let the young man depart, and commanded *him,* "Tell no one that you have revealed these things to me."

G-d warned him through this person that there were forty men who were fasting until they would see Paul dead. It looks to me like the young man's message was intercepted and never reached Paul. Help me someone…

Acts 23:29 - I found out that he was accused concerning questions of their law, but had nothing charged against him deserving of death or chains.

Honest evaluation.

Acts 24:19 - They ought to have been here before you to object if they had anything against me.

Paul defended his worship in Jerusalem, his offering to his nation of Judea and felt that the only objection would be that he believed in the resurrection of the dead.

Acts 24:23 - So he commanded the centurion to keep Paul and to let *him* have liberty, and told him not to forbid any of his friends to provide for or visit him.

This is heartwarming since he's suffered plenty up to now.

Acts 24:25-26 - Now as he reasoned about righteousness, self-control, and the judgment to come, Felix was afraid and answered, "Go away for now; when I have a convenient time I will call for you." 26 Meanwhile he also hoped that money would be given him by Paul, [NU omits that he might release him] that he might release him. Therefore he sent for him more often and conversed with him.

Like today, "bribery" is a way.

Acts 25:1 - Now when Festus had come to the province, after three days he went up from Caesarea to Jerusalem.

In Jerusalem some mean Jewish leaders told Festus nasty things about Paul. They asked for him to be brought to Jerusalem but their intent was to kill him on the way. Their plan was frustrated.

Acts 26:6 - And now I stand and am judged for the hope of the promise made by God to our fathers.

Festus was impressed and asked if he'd be willing to go to Jerusalem, but he appealed to Caesar and to Caesar in Rome he would go.

Acts 26:8 - Why should it be thought incredible by you that God raises the dead?

Excellent question!

Acts 26:17-18 - I will [rescue] deliver you from the *Jewish* people, as well as *from* the Gentiles, to whom I [NU, M omit now] now send you, [18] to open their eyes, *in order* to turn *them* from darkness to light, and *from* the power of Satan to God, that they may receive forgiveness of sins and an inheritance among those who are sanctified[set apart] by faith in Me.'

This is a beautiful testimony in a nutshell. Isn't it reassuring that even if we have hardly anything of this world's goods, we have an inheritance which is eternal and will not be stolen from us.

Acts 26:24 - Now as he thus made his defense, Festus said with a loud voice, "Paul, you are beside yourself! Much learning is driving you mad!"

A typical reaction of one who doesn't believe in the supernatural.

Acts 26:28 - Then Agrippa said to Paul, "You almost persuade me to become a Christian."

This is a famous quote. Only G-d knows if we'll see Agrippa in the next world.

Acts 26:31 - and when they had gone aside, they talked among themselves, saying, "This man is doing nothing deserving of death or chains."

They're thinking reasonably.

Acts 27:3 - And the next *day* we landed at Sidon. And Julius treated Paul kindly and gave *him* liberty to go to his friends and receive care.

Wonderful.

Acts 27:11 - Nevertheless the centurion was more persuaded by the helmsman and the owner of the ship than by the things spoken by Paul.

Why should they have listened since they're the "experts!"

Acts 27:22 - And now I urge you to take [courage]heart, for there will be no loss of life among you, but only of the ship.

G-d's mercy despite not being willing to listen to Paul's G-d-given wisdom

Acts 27:35 - And when he had said these things, he took bread and gave thanks to God in the presence of them all; and when he had broken *it* he began to eat.

They were an orderly bunch not breaking into the food like savages. PTL they could FINALLY eat.

Acts 28:2 - And the natives[barbarians] showed us unusual kindness; for they kindled a fire and made us all welcome, because of the rain that was falling and because of the cold.

"Unusual" kindness. This is noteworthy.

Acts 28:6 - However, they were expecting that he would swell up or suddenly fall down dead. But after they had looked for a long time and saw no harm come to him, they changed their minds and said that he was a god.

Tangible truth that G-d's promise to the disciples was in effect from Luke 10:19 Behold, I give you the authority to trample on serpents and scorpions, and over all the power of the enemy, and nothing shall by any means hurt you.

Acts 28:9-10 - So when this was done, the rest of those on the island who had diseases also came and were healed. 10 They also honored us in many ways; and when we departed, they provided such things as were necessary.

It couldn't have been a better outcome for a bunch of shipwrecked folks.

Acts 28:20 - For this reason therefore I have called for you, to see *you* and speak with *you,* because for the hope of Israel I am bound with this chain."

Paul reached out to the Jewish leaders in Rome and wished to speak with them. He testified of the kingdom of G-d, persuading them concerning Jesus from both the Law of Moses and the Prophets, from morning till evening. He quoted from Isaiah 6:9-10 9 And He said, "Go, and tell this people:

> 'Keep on hearing, but do not understand;
> Keep on seeing, but do not perceive.'
>
> 10 "Make the heart of this people dull,
> And their ears heavy,
> And shut their eyes;
> Lest they see with their eyes,
> And hear with their ears,
> And understand with their heart,
> And return and be healed."

Some of them disputed among themselves. He also said that the salvation of G-d has been sent to the Gentiles, and they will hear it!" Do we realize that because of so many believing Gentiles around the world today, that Isaiah had prophesied this and Paul had preached Isaiah?

Acts 28:30 - Then Paul dwelt two whole years in his own rented house, and received all who came to him,

He received ALL – would we do the same?

Romans 1:24 - Therefore God also gave them up to uncleanness, in the lusts of their hearts, to dishonor their bodies among themselves,

Description of our world in 2021.

Romans 1:32 - who, knowing the righteous judgment of God, that those who practice such things are deserving of death, not only do the same but also approve of those who practice them.

Just because they, themselves, don't practice them, it's as bad to APPROVE of those who practice them.

"PROOF OF HEALING" BOOKS

The Happiest People on Earth, *Living a Life of Fire*, *Holiness and Healing* (by Dan Bohi and Dr Rob McCorkle), *Harvest Glory: I Ask for the Nations* (by Ruth Ward Heflin), *A Foretaste of Glory Divine* (by Jane Lowder and Harold McDougal).

ADDITIONAL READING AT HOME

Since one needs to take it easy back home, apart from the minor effort when it comes to exercising for a while daily, what can one do but read? The books I read when back home were *One Divine Moment, Confronting radicals, What are the Odds?, Fault Line, Releasing Prophetic Destiny, Holiness and Healing, Intercessory Prayer, Authority in Prayer, Shaping History – Prayer and Fasting, with All Your Heart, Conquering the Chaos in Your Mind, The Oracle, The Love Languages of God, The Rock, the Road and the Rabbi, A Handbook to Marriage, Reset: Jesus Changes Everything, Enemies and Allies, A Foretaste of Glory Divine, The Christian Left, and Jeremiah's last Call.*

LOOKING BACK

Now I'm 75. I've travelled a road veering to the side of faith healing at times, and to the other side of trusting competent doctors, who possess G-d's wisdom (even if they don't give Him credit!). The Pentecostals had a great impact on me in Jerusalem. I can say that despite the "high" I experienced in the Bible school in England, together with the valuable teaching I received the following summer in France in the Child Evangelism course didn't compare with what awaited me in Jerusalem. I do thank the Lord for CEF since, although by law we're forbidden to witness to minors in Israel, no one prevented from teaching my own children. I taught them Bible and missionary stories. When I no longer needed the materials, I passed them on to a daughter-in-law who has been using them since they're teaching many believing children. My son also teaches. In fact, three out of my four children have taught children in their lifetimes.

The Jerusalem experience put me on an even keel. In the USA I was fervent and even joined outreach teams. I joined Campus Crusade for Christ and went witnessing on the beach at spring break. I had results. I was encouraged. I would attend many summer conferences and weekend conferences. Still, there were those "down" periods. After my Holy Spirit experience I felt that I was no longer dependent on a certain conference, retreat or special speaker to prop me up. After attending the yearly ICEJ Feast of Tabernacles, I felt a fresh injection of encouragement or even power from the great teaching there. My children also gained much from their children's sessions. Once my daughter told me she had nice dreams afterwards. The music would stay in my mind and heart for a few days following. I say this because it was missing for two years due to the covid-19 pandemic. I haven't lost my faith as a result of not being in Jerusalem or being in our regular congregation. I haven't lost my faith as a result of having to watch zoom calls for a year.

I would like to put in a plug for the WorldPrayerNetwork, my new "family." Dr. Jim Garlow, Mario Bramnick and Adam W. Schindler hosted a prayer call the day after President Biden was elected. It was called, "Global Prayer for U.S. Election Integrity." Their purpose was to PRAY that righteousness, justice, truth and holiness would prevail in the land (the USA). They even state this before every call. They have the shofar played also before each call. I like this since it's like, "WAKE UP, EVERYONE!" I'm happy to report that in the USA many have awakened. I'm seeing and understanding that not only did Jim Garlow leave a pastorate of many years, but Lance Wallnau, whom I've been following for years (but not lately) also left a pastorate. Their ministries point out that church folks need to be entering ALL of the seven spheres of influence in our society, including and especially government. Due to the missing Christian voice in politics in the USA, the evil laws were made. Now they're trying desperately to undo them and bring America back to her calling by G-d to be a light on a hill. The founding fathers were Christian but evil people are coming in and changing history. They want little children to think that there was too much bad stuff, like black slavery, and they don't see the good things; namely the freedom of speech, religion, and other things. In fact, these basic freedoms we see are under attack. It should be a great concern to G-d's people especially.

There were 27 calls and then they changed the name to WorldPrayerNetwork. Sadly after a particular broadcast about the vaccines, they were pushed off of youtube. They can be found on Facebook, Vimeo, and their own WPN network. If I know anything about the USA, it's thanks to the information I have received from over 100 calls. On the 50th call on July 25th, Dan Bohi talked about divine healing. As I was listening, knowing that he ministers to thousands and thousands of people and many of whom have been healed, I prayed for my own post-surgery healing. I was in terrible pain. My son was going to purchase some narcotic med for me. He was going out the door but I phoned and stopped him. The Lord eased the pain and since those two weeks of recovery in the hospital I have used only lesser meds. This was a great victory.

Bill Gothard came to Long Beach, California to do his series on "Basic Youth Conflicts", and folks would drive for miles to hear him. We had a thick notebook with lots of great teaching. I think this was in the 1960's. He advocated fasting once a week. Strangely enough, the Lord had shown me a year earlier the blessing of fasting. I HAD read about it in a book by Malla Moe. She was a Norwegian missionary to Africa. To this day from the 70's I have fasted at last once a week. In my pension years I go two days a week since I'm sitting for hours at the computer. The Lord always shows me from the scriptures when to end a fast. I was so grieved about the situation in the states I went on an every-other-day fast for five months. I survived. Then I did Esther fasts for the first time every time one of those crucial dates came up in the USA. It wasn't so easy going without water but I mostly stayed at home. I could sleep when needed. I did four of them and another in the process of writing this book (FINALLY!). The Lord showed me that I could finish this fast early by about 12 hours since most of the book had been completed. The brain becomes more focused. FOOD is such a big part of our lives and such a distraction even when one eats simple, healthy foods which don't take lots of preparation.

Some people reading this book are aware that some so-called, divine healers aren't really from G-d. You can even quote the scripture. People have been healed in a meeting and died shortly afterwards. What was wrong? To answer this question I'll only remind you of the ten lepers whom Yeshua healed. Only one came back to thank Him. They were also supposed to go to the priest. What if they didn't? Would their leprosy return? I'm not able to answer these questions. One sound Bible teacher says that after we're healed we need to give testimony of our healing and thereby be strengthened. If a non-churched person is healed, he/she should surely seek out like-minded believers so they grow in their faith.

I personally feel that if a person with severe health issues claims to have been healed, they need to do whatever they can, in addition, so as not to tempt the Lord. If the person is obese, they need to work on the problem. I also strongly recommend fasting to everyone unless it's strongly prohibited. Not only will it draw you closer to Yeshua, it will surprise you how much time you have to get things done which you hadn't gotten to. It's the best remedy for being alert during exams or at work if you're expecting an unusually busy day.

Do I regret having a knee replacement? Of course not. My husband and I both visited our son's family in Germany before the pandemic. Every day I was there I needed to take a strong medicine called Arcoxia in order to walk. Then for our 40th anniversary we traveled to southwestern Italy. It was a great trip with a group. Again, every day I needed to take this med which can affect the liver. After the covid-19 shutdowns I hope and pray that we can take more trips abroad together. I have heard many positive reports about those who did the knee replacement and only one negative one. The particular person who was dissatisfied had an infection when in the hospital. I anticipate walking a lot and even running!

If someone with osteoporosis, particularly an older person like me, doesn't believe bones can improve, I report to you that my last test showed 12% and 9% improvement. I still take a once-a-week pill called Fosavance. Even though the bones improved, it didn't relate to the knee cartilage problem, therefore the surgery was necessary. The extreme fasting which I did was after the test so I await results later on. The bone density test is done only every three years. Fasting does not make ones bones worse. In Isaiah 58:6-12 we read,

> "*Is* this not the fast that I have chosen:
> To loose the bonds of wickedness,

To undo the [Lit. bonds of the yoke] heavy burdens,
To let the oppressed go free,
And that you break every yoke?
7 *Is it* not to share your bread with the hungry,
And that you bring to your house the poor
who are [wandering] cast out;
When you see the naked, that you cover him,
And not hide yourself from your own flesh?
8 Then your light shall break forth like the
morning,
Your healing shall spring forth speedily,
And your righteousness shall go before you;
The glory of the LORD shall be your rear guard.
9 Then you shall call, and the LORD will answer;
You shall cry, and He will say, 'Here I *am.*'
"If you take away the yoke from your midst,
The [Lit. sending out of] pointing of the finger, and
speaking wickedness,
10 *If* you extend your soul to the hungry
And satisfy the afflicted soul,
Then your light shall dawn in the darkness,
And your [Or gloom] darkness shall *be* as the noonday.
11 The LORD will guide you continually,
And satisfy your soul in drought,
And strengthen your bones;
You shall be like a watered garden,
And like a spring of water, whose waters do
not fail.

[12] Those from among you
Shall build the old waste places;
You shall raise up the foundations of many generations;
And you shall be called the Repairer of the Breach,
The Restorer of [Lit. Paths] Streets to Dwell In.

Note especially verse 11.

CONCLUSION

If anyone reading this book has decided it's OK to have a surgical knee replacement, I have succeeded. If someone has been blessed with my insights into the various scriptures which the Lord underlined in my mind during my hospital stay, I have succeeded. If someone has understood how the supernatural can still occur, and does, as opposed to the thinking of many G-d fearing and biblical folks, I will have succeeded. I felt that the Lord wanted me to write this book. Had I not taken any notes throughout these past months, there would not be a book, of course. I had some "dry bones" on which I could put some flesh.

Oral Roberts decided to build a hospital near the campus of the university where faith healing was taught. Does this seem strange to you? Dr. Paul Enenche, a trained medical doctor, directs healing services. Does one contradict the other? For me there is no contradiction.

My apologies if I left out someone you felt should have been included. You may write me at live26isr@yahoo.com. Your comments, criticisms, testimonies, etc. are welcome.

Just in time before final publishing of this book, I'm happy to report that WPN is back on YouTube.

I wish everyone good health and joy in Yeshua, who makes life worth living. Take care of yourselves, brothers and sisters, and most of all, "let the Word dwell in you richly" (Colossians 3:16).

BIBLIOGRAPHY

Charles Clarke, *Pioneers of Revival*, Logos International, Plainfield, NJ, 1971.

https://www.biblegateway.com New King James Version for the Bible texts.

M =Mounce Reverse Interlinear New Testament (MOUNCE)

https://en.wikipedia.org/wiki/Atlantic_slave_trade

https://en.wikipedia.org/wiki/Albert_Benjamin_Simpson (11.9.18)

https://en.wikipedia.org/wiki/Maria_Woodworth-Etter (13.2.18)

https://en.wikipedia.org/wiki/Alexander_Boddy (14.2.18)

https://en.wikipedia.org/wiki/Smith_Wigglesworth

https://en.wikipedia.org/wiki/Thomas_Ball_Barratt (8 September 2021)

https://en.wikipedia.org/wiki/John_G._Lake (28.9.18)

https://en.wikipedia.org/wiki/Stanley_Frodsham (6 July 2021)

https://sites.google.com/view/adpcm/e-h-top-page/glover-kelso-r

https://en.wikipedia.org/wiki/Lewi_Pethrus (21 September 2021)

https://healingandrevival.com/BioCSPrice.htm

https://en.wikipedia.org/wiki/Aimee_Semple_McPherson

https://news.ag.org/features/this-week-in-ag-history-july-11-1942 (John Peter Kolenda)

https://en.wikipedia.org/wiki/James_Gordon_Lindsay (3.9.18)

https://en.wikipedia.org/wiki/Kathryn_Kuhlman (27.9.18)

https://en.wikipedia.org/wiki/A._A._Allen (2.11.21)

https://revival-books.com/products/visions-of-heaven-hell-and-the-cross-fox

https://www.araratchurch.com/about-us (Bishop Harry A. Mushegan)

https://en.wikipedia.org/wiki/Oral_Roberts (29.9.18)

https://lrm1948.blogspot.com/2008/12/charlotte-bakers-prophetic-parables.html

https://godswordtowomen.org/shaw.htm

http://www.sandornemeth.com/faith-church/confession-of-faith/gifts-holy-spirit

ACKNOWLEDGMENTS

Many thanks to the very efficient JETLAUNCH team; Chris O'Byrne, Debbie O'Byrne, and Teri Kojetin. Special thanks to Dvora Hemstreet who helped me with all of my books. She also did the knee replacement operation and while still recovering was willing to help. Last, but not least, I am blessed beyond words with the support of my husband, Michael, my husband of 42 ½ years, not only during the post-surgery period, but while preparing this book.

Made in the USA
Monee, IL
04 November 2026

67380833R00105